Robert,
Thanks for tell —
your story, & thank you
for the book exchange.

11/20/15

INVISIBLE

PTSD'S STEALTH ATTACK
ON A VIETNAM WAR VETERAN

Welcome home;
Peace; Bill Blaylock

William J. Blaylock

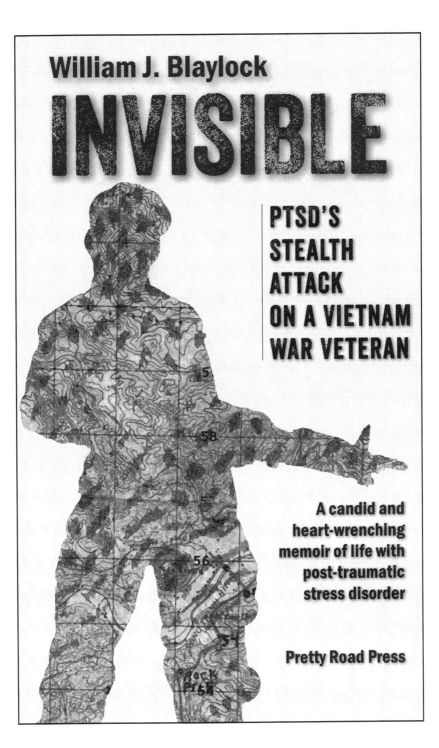

William J. Blaylock

INVISIBLE

PTSD'S STEALTH ATTACK ON A VIETNAM WAR VETERAN

A candid and heart-wrenching memoir of life with post-traumatic stress disorder

Pretty Road Press

Invisible:
   PTSD's Stealth Attack on a Vietnam Veteran,
   a Candid and Heart-Wrenching Memoir
   of Life with Post-Traumatic Stress Disorder

Published by
Pretty Road Press
P.O. Box 273
Folsom, California 95763
www.PrettyRoadPress.com

© 2013, Pretty Road Press

Printed in the United States of America

ISBN 978-0-9826014-6-4

17 16 15 14   5 4 3 2

To all known and unknown warriors of the Vietnam War, and also to the warriors of all wars.

Specifically, I dedicate this book to:

Sgt. Mjr. Sam L. Topps
Sgt. Leonard Bruski
Spc. 4 Dennis Ramsey
Sgt. Cuba C. Wright
Spc. 4 Anthony Lee
Spc. 4 "Shorty" Thomas
Spc. 4 Terry Holmes
Sgt. "Zique" McHenry
The dead and injured marines on Highway 9
The marine with his severed right hand
Lan, the Vietnamese boy
My fellow PTSD group members:
Harry "Bubba" St. John
Andy "Taco" Martinez
Gary "Tank" Duncan
Don "Doc" Dali
Jim "Bart" Bartholomew
Skip "Cowboy"/"Crazy Man" Petit
Tony "Korea" Trejo

And to all my known, and unknown "Brothers in Arms"

Invisible

Acknowledgments

I thank my wife Betty, son John, daughter Tiffany, granddaughter Dahlia, and all my family, friends, doctors, and counselors, whom I hope I have not embarrassed or alienated by including them in my writing.

I also thank and express my great appreciation to Catherine Close, my writing coach. Without her support and knowledge, this work and memoir would not have been completed. Thank you, Catherine.

Finally, I thank Pretty Road Press for picking up my book and taking it to market.

Invisible

Foreword

The book you hold is not a medical textbook, nor is it a war story. It is Bill Blaylock's personal story of his journey to discover what caused him to suffer needlessly from an injury that, until very recently, was often misdiagnosed. It is still misunderstood. I learned from this book what post-traumatic stress disorder (PTSD) really is and how it can affect everyone — not just those who have been physically injured in combat operations. Bill shares his struggles through much of his post-Vietnam adult life without ever realizing that he had been injured by his experience in Vietnam. He reveals how it took a friend, who also had PTSD, to convince him that he, too, was injured and that he needed to seek medical help if he was ever going to recover.

When Bill asked me to write the Foreword to his book, Invisible, PTSD's Stealth Attack on a Vietnam War Veteran, I was honored and perplexed. Honored because he wanted my opinion on a subject I knew little about and perplexed for the same reason. I first met Bill and his wife Betty at our church. We worked together at various times and served together periodically at Sunday services, but I did not know much about his background. He took his responsibilities seriously and always had a smile on his face. Then one day he asked if I would read and comment on a book he had written.

One evening a few days later, I began to read Bill's manuscript thinking that it would take me several days to be able to have enough time to read the entire manuscript. I finished reading Bill's story that same evening—I simply could not put it down.

The military life is one I know well, but I must admit I have limited knowledge of PTSD and no personal experience. I spent thirty-three years in service, starting with three years as a seaman in the U.S. Navy Reserve and then thirty years in U.S. Air Force Logistics. I am not a pilot, and while I was in Vietnam on a number of occasions for temporary duty, I was always on an airbase and never experienced combat. When I was in Thailand for a one-year tour at Nakhom Phanom RTAFB, it was near the end of the Vietnam War. We worked seven days a week through the evacuation of Phenom Penh and Saigon, and supporting the air force CH-53 and HH-53 helicopters that flew marines to Koh Tang Island in rescue of the crew from the SS Mayaguez, but again, I was not personally involved in the combat operations.

We continue to learn from the thousands of military men and women who have served one or more tours of duty in Iraq and Afghanistan and those who served in all the military operations before. PTSD is a silent injury that most do not want to speak about. Bill's personal story lifts the cloak of silence and fear from this seemingly invisible injury. He helps us realize that it isn't just combat that can injure people's psyche with the debilitating effects of PTSD, it can be any number of other traumatic events that any one of us can experience.

Bill's story is a valuable contribution toward our efforts to understand PTSD. I hope this book will be used by families and anyone who might have this terrible condition, so that they can know that they are not alone and that they can get help to deal with it.

I thank Bill for having the courage to tell his story in Invisible, PTSD's Stealth Attack on a Vietnam War Veteran.

James W. Hopp
Major General, USAF (Retired)
Sacramento, California

Invisible

Preface

Most of the time, we do not even know anything is wrong. We just want to get away from people. We are nervous and on edge. We are always in a state of hyper-vigilance and never fully trust anyone. We will not allow anyone to get too close to us. We employ emotional numbing because our loss will be too painful.

When we came home, we had plans about how great everything was going to be. Maybe we were going to buy a car or go back to school. Maybe we were just going to make love without stopping for days without end. But it wasn't that way at all. Sure, our families were glad to have us back home, but they had their own plans for our return. And somehow the two didn't seem to match. Then there is the slightly noticeable fact (to others) that we were not quite the same guy we were when we left.

Now is when the symptoms start to show. If we are lucky enough to have a job waiting for us or something productive to do, we start trying to suppress our thoughts and emotions because we have always been told to man-up. I'm not saying that is a bad thing; it's actually what allows us to stay focused for a while, pushing that stuff back in our mind to a place where it won't bother us.

Then a time comes, as with so many Vietnam veterans, when life slows down. We suddenly have time to reflect. The anxiety and emotion soon return to the forefront of our minds, and then intrude into the very fabric of our lives.

I sincerely hope that our next generation of warriors will not wait forty years to seek the aid and professional attention of Vet Centers and Veterans Administration medical facilities.

Have you heard these words?

"I need a drink."

"I need to get away from here."

"I hate being around all these people."

"Leave me alone."

"Nothing's the matter; just don't bug me."

"I'm out of here."

Have you said these words to someone you know or love, but can't tell them what you really want and need to say? Have you said them to your family? Maybe you've said something like this to your parents, wives, children, girlfriends, or employers. I made these relationships plural because I have had several of each. We are reactive to our depression, hyper-vigilance, anger, and other symptoms of PTSD that cause us to be frequently divorced, fired, and self-medicated with alcohols and or drugs. Everyone wants and needs personal relationships, but for most of us with PTSD, they are just too difficult to maintain. We back away from people, and stay numb to personal relations.

Some came home with missing fingers, hands, arms, feet, and legs, but for the wounded mind, there is no compassion or understanding. "What's your problem?" someone asks, or says, "Get over it." They are the responses of many people who cannot see the outward signs of injury for which war is responsible.

PTSD is called a disorder. Even its name is negative. It leaves the patient feeling ashamed. Outsiders think it does not actually exist. Disorder is and of itself a derogatory word. I think most people believe that if a person is said to have a condition or disorder, they are considered to be just a little outside of the normal. It does mean that something is wrong, or there is an illness, but it does not give the respect of an injury that post-traumatic stress deserves. Yes, there is something wrong, but if the disorder were replaced with a visible injury, it would indicate to everyone that there is, indeed, a wound, or injury and a need for healing. It wouldn't be invisible. It is this stealthy malady that psychologists and psychiatrists at Veteran Centers and Veterans Administration mental health facilities all across the United States attempt to address.

THIS BOOK IS ABOUT MY EXPERIENCE as a Vietnam veteran and how it affected my life.

I do not seek sympathy in the course of telling my story. In fact, putting my life on paper was very difficult to do. My reason for writing this book is to let people know what I experienced while serving in Vietnam. Hopefully, it will help others recognize their own traumas. Writing this book has helped heal my own wounds, and I recommend writing to anyone who doesn't want to talk or who cannot talk about what they are thinking and feeling.

TO HELP UNDERSTAND WHAT PTSD is, and how it affects a person, I begin by defining it:

Post-traumatic stress disorder (PTSD) is an anxiety disorder that can occur after you have been through a traumatic event. A traumatic event is something horrible and scary that you see or that happens to you. During this type of event, you think that your life or others' lives are in danger. You may feel afraid or feel that you have no control over what is happening.

Anyone who has gone through a life-threatening event can develop PTSD. Traumatic events can include:

- Combat or military exposure
- Child sexual or physical abuse
- Terrorist attacks
- Sexual or physical assault
- Serious accidents, such as a car wreck
- Natural disasters, such as a fire, hurricane, flood, or earthquake.

After the event, you may feel scared, confused, or angry. If these feelings don't go away or if they get worse, you may have PTSD. These symptoms may disrupt your life, making it hard to continue with your daily activities, according to the U.S. Department of Veterans Affairs.

PTSD can result from many different traumas, from traffic accidents, natural disasters, and crime. This book is about my experience of PTSD caused by war.

My goal for this book is to help others to understand PTSD and its effects, both physical and mental, caused by trauma. Trauma happens to people every day and everywhere in our lives. We are involved in and witness brutal, death-causing traffic accidents; we have losses and experience the death of parents, loved ones, friends, and family. Some are assaulted, and more specific to women, some suffer the brutal trauma of rape—all to which we feel powerless and have no control over.

THE PLACES IN THIS BOOK ARE REAL. However, some names have been changed or left out to protect their anonymity. The actions told in *Invisible: PTSD's Stealth Attack on a Vietnam War Veteran* are real, although places, dates, times, and order of events may have been changed. These events are drawn out of my own experience and shared to the best of my remembrance. Most conversations depicted are reconstructed from my best recollection. If there are inaccuracies, they are mine, and mine alone.

IT TOOK OUR MILITARY AND GOVERNMENT a long time to recognize and admit this complex and extensive problem, subsequent to any military action or war. Nevertheless, at last, through many years of diligent pressure by my fellow veterans, there is recognition and now true professional help.

Thank you to the people and government of the United States of America. Thank you also Vet Centers and the Veterans Administration for your network of medical centers and hospitals to care for veterans in need.

1

Rockpile, Vietnam: 1968

Straining to look over my left shoulder, I see two F-4 Phantoms making their approach to drop napalm and high explosive ordinance from the pylons beneath their wings. They dive down from their lofty altitude in the clear blue sky toward my location on the ground. I lose sight of them as they thread their way and skim just above the top of the mountainous jungle canopy, injecting their venomous destruction. Immediately after the drop, they climb back to the sky, breaking left and right respectively to evade enemy fire. They regroup and return to deliver more high-explosive bombs to help subdue the attacking enemy force. I pray to myself that none of our marines are so far from the road as to have been hit by the napalm and shrapnel from the high-explosive ordinance. The shock waves of the bombs shake my Duster, a tracked, open-turret tank with two 40-mm guns. The heat burns against the left side of my face, and then I fight to breathe as the napalm sucks oxygen from the air feeding its explosive inferno of fire.

We've been called to assist a company of marines who have been pinned down and taking fire from both sides of the road in an ambush at a mountain ravine on Highway 9, east of our location at the Rockpile. The river flows on my left, and the ravine lies on my right. The area is full of vegetation. Up the ravine and across the river onto the other side, the ground gives rise to dense trees and brush. A shallow ditch parallels the ravine side of the road, probably made when the road was graded. It fails to provide much protection from the enemy fire spraying down on us. Our extra firepower is needed for a platoon of marines to rescue the wounded and retrieve the dead.

Yelling into the radio, the lieutenant orders, "Drive in there firing. Shoot everything that moves. Kill those little bastards."

"Oh shit, here we go," I think, firing as many rounds as possible as we move forward to allow the marines to regroup and begin an assault.

We are the lead track assigned the right side, firing up into the ravine, while the other Duster takes the left, firing on the area between the road and the river that has just been napalmed and bombed by the U.S. Air Force F-4 Phantoms.

Lee, the driver, moves us into the kill zone with bodies of marines, dead and alive, still on the road ahead. Marines are crouched low and close to the side of the Duster, providing them protection on their blind side. My buddy Len fires the M60 mounted on the back of the turret, and the marines return fire with their M16 and M79 grenade launchers as we drive in. I pray, "Dear God, let the marines beside us move the bodies away from the path of our tracks before Lee has to drive over them to get us into firing position."

The enemy rains down fire as we move into position. Rounds strike our Duster and the ground around us. Miraculously none of us have been hit. We fire back, doing our job. Only seconds have passed since we started the barrage. I fire our 40-mm guns as fast as possible, when suddenly the enemy fire stops. We continue to fire at everything, so they won't have a chance to rise up and resume their attack. We spray rounds all over the ravine, not knowing the exact enemy positions. The other Duster protects our back, firing on the other side of the road, as we each protect the other.

Some of the injured marines are loaded onto the sides of the Dusters to take them back down the road to a helicopter landing zone, known as the LZ, where they can be evacuated to a hospital. A wounded marine, slung in his own poncho, is lifted up on the side for transport.

Len and I hold the marine in the poncho while we drive to the LZ. His helmet falls off as he is lifted up, and his light brown hair is the only thing not masked in mud. He's covered with drying mud and blood—his own blood and this dammed red mud of Vietnam, coagulating together. I can't tell where the mud stops and his blood begins. Two empty morphine syringes are pinned to his left collar.

Entry wounds cover his body: his legs, arms, and face—everywhere except where his flak vest prevented any more torso wounds. The vest is riddled with tears, exposing its own mangled interior fabric where it has been hit and ripped open. I see the whites of his eyes. When he speaks to us, I see his teeth, bright-white, each one outlined with red blood and saliva in stark contrast against his filthy face

I wonder, "What the hell was he hit with to have so many damned entry wounds—a grenade, mine, or what?"

A corpsman presses bandages under his clothing to stop the bleeding, but he is still oozing fresh blood everywhere. The two empty morphine dispensers attached to his collar fall against his neck each time he moves.

I still hear shooting back in the ravine as marines continue to pursue the enemy. The noise level is so intense it is difficult to concentrate. It is loud with gunfire and yelling. They combine with the noise of the motor, along with the piercing, squeaking sound of grinding metal from the tracks on our Duster. Smoke fills the burning jungle where napalm has hit. The air smells thick with gunpowder. The burning scent of the fight fills my nostrils. It sears my nose! The smell is reminiscent of a Fourth of July fireworks show back home, yet so different.

Then, amid all the commotion, everything goes silent, as though I have suddenly gone deaf. In the quiet, almost in slow motion, the muddy, bloody marine raises his right arm to show Len and me that his right hand remains barely attached, hanging only by skin at his wrist. Bone and flesh plainly expose themselves, but no blood drips. A tourniquet on his arm stops the flow. Looking up at us with a snicker of a smile on his lips and with a slight laugh in his voice, he tells us, "I guess I'll have to learn how to jack off with my left hand!"

As suddenly as they stopped, the sounds of the war return, and we move backward down the dirt road to a freshly blown LZ.

I CANNOT HOLD BACK THE MEMORY or the tears. I am not in Vietnam, and it is not 1968. It is November, 2010. I am sitting at my home computer, looking at the country of Vietnam on Google Earth.

"How long have I been out, back there in my mind?" I wonder. Looking at the clock on the wall, I realize it has only been seconds, maybe minutes. My flashbacks are like dreams. Scenes that took minutes and hours in real time only take seconds to replay in my mind.

"When is this shit going to stop?"

2

With a Friend's Help

October 26, 2006. With my friend Sam's encouragement, I contacted the Sacramento Vet Center, a branch of the Veterans Administration, and found my way to help. I discovered the counseling sessions were not stressful. In fact, they usually left me feeling good. However, the more I talked, the more I began to remember. I had worked so hard to forget and suppress my thoughts, fears, and emotions of Vietnam, filing them away into deep folders I had created for myself over forty years. Now, the more I talked and thought about my experience, the more details I remembered. Counseling took place only once a month, which gave me plenty of time to reflect between sessions.

When first asked by my Vet Center counselor if I wanted to file a claim for post-traumatic stress disorder, commonly referred to as PTSD, I thought it sounded rather greedy on my part, and a somewhat curious first question on her part. I told my counselor, "No, I just want to get better and not feel so depressed and anxious around people." Counseling continued for six months until I realized I didn't really feel different. In retrospect, I don't know why I thought that I should feel anything after counseling, talking, remembering, and calling it all back up. I distinctly recall one of my last sessions at the Vet Center; I got to my car to leave and turned on the radio. It was April 16, 2007. The announcer delivered news that a shooter had killed thirty-two and wounded twenty-five people on the Virginia Tech campus. I couldn't take it any longer; I just sat there and cried.

At work one day, a feeling came over me for no apparent reason; it made me want to cry. I went to the only place there was for privacy to compose myself: the men's room. After a few minutes, I was able to return to work. Over the next several months, this behavior became a pattern. If I took more than a couple minutes to collect myself, I would try to disguise the situation by spraying some air freshener before leaving the room.

I could still force myself to go places with my wife where many people were present, but I would always find a place to hang out where I could be by myself, where there was also an easy escape route for a quick departure if necessary.

Months passed before I contacted the Veterans Administration mental health clinic that the Vet Center counselor had recommended. At the clinic, I spoke with an interviewer who submitted paperwork for me to follow up on so that I could get an appointment with a psychiatrist.

Although Vietnam was forty years gone, I remained closed with my thoughts and feelings, unable to open up to anyone. I was certainly not going to open myself to a stranger. I needed to validate a person before telling them anything personal. Even me talking to fellow vets required knowing that their combat experience would allow them to understand what I might reveal about myself.

The VA Mental Health Department prepared an appointment for me with a psychiatrist I named simply Dr. Jack. He asked questions to help me share experiences and feelings held so close for so long. It actually took several sessions for me to finally tell him what I thought were my real fears and feelings. His schedule only allowed for thirty-minute appointments, but by paying close attention, he made me feel that I could trust him and that he believed what I was saying. He helped me cope with my emotions when they hit me at work. He taught me a meditation technique that helped me to relax and compose myself faster. I learned to go to my private place. I would sit or stand, concentrating on one simple thing, my breathing. I would just concentrate on slow, long, deep breaths.

"Try to think only about your breathing," he told me. "It takes some practice, but you can learn to focus your thoughts on that simple life task, and pretty soon all other thoughts and frustrations are gone."

Sometimes it worked and sometimes it failed.

Dr. Jack suggested I attend a group session that would be soon starting to inform and assist vets with PTSD. I signed up for an eleven-week session. Immediately, the class pointed out and made me aware of actions and conditions that I had been experiencing over the last forty years. They were the often-invisible symptoms of PTSD. I was blind to the wounds PTSD had inflicted. I failed to connect my experiences, feelings and behavior to PTSD, past experience or trauma.

The doctors explained that my frustration and anxiety could become more acute, particularly at an older age, as life slows down and the mind has more time to remember. Events like 9/11 and wars in Kuwait, Iraq, and Afghanistan all contributed to ignite an explosion of traumatic emotion in me and most of the others attending the session. Soon I realized I was not the only person to get up from bed each night to check the perimeter or to suffer reoccurring nightmares and flashbacks. The program turned out to be an informative and rewarding experience. After completion of the initial eleven-week course, we enjoyed the opportunity to sign up for a much more intensive weekly group session that would last about six months. It would make a difference.

The group consisted of nine vets and a psychiatrist. Our group facilitator kept us on track, but we freely expressed what we thought, felt, and feared—in the safety and comfort of our small group. The psychiatrist encouraged us to write a letter, offering a confession, apology, or information to address our trauma. Then we would safely read our letters to the group. The final meeting of the group concluded with a ceremonial disposal of all letters written. While similar groups had ceremonially burned their letters, our group willed them to two VA psychologists so they could be used to help others, whether they became published, analyzed, or read by other hurting veterans. I soaked up the help provided by the group and continued my daily routine and work.

THREE WOMEN CAME INTO THE STORE where I worked. They were small in stature and wore medium-gray pajama-type pants covered with the traditional, long over-garment. Two wore small skullcaps. The third wore a large-brimmed, pointed hat with a chinstrap like the ones Vietnamese farmers wore in their fields.

Their presence enraged me. I had to leave the store and go outside. I asked one of the other employees to cover for me while the women were in the building. I paced, overcome by cold sweats, racing heart, and rapid breath. The women hadn't asked for help; they were just wandering around the store looking at things. Maybe they didn't speak English well enough or at all. I learned that they spent about fifteen minutes shopping, then left without buying anything.

Because each of them wore all gray, I surmised they might be nuns. I didn't know of any Buddhist temples in the area, so I had no idea where they might have come from, but I made an association. They wore the only clothing I saw worn in Vietnam: these same outfits, either all black or, sometimes, a white top with black pajamas.

Despite the war's distance, the experience at the store upset me. It told me I had not yet been able to get past the deep-seated intolerance I harbored for these people.

The more I reflected on the occurrence, the more I noticed that, not only had I become unable to function in my duties for fifteen minutes or more, but I was also unable to completely concentrate for several hours. All the time I spent outside pacing, I kept telling myself there was nothing to be afraid of; I was being silly. I felt no fear of them, exactly. Instead, I was afraid of my own actions. What would I do if I lost my temper?

At the end of the day, I was completely exhausted. I got home that evening and poured myself three fingers of Jim Beam. I sat in a quiet place for a half-hour before I could tell my wife about what had happened.

On that occasion, I had the presence of mind to remove myself from the threat. What would I do if it ever happened again?

At my next PTSD group meeting, I shared my thoughts. The consensus of the group was that I had handled the situation as well as could be expected. Everyone agreed that, had they not been dressed in that typical Vietnamese clothing, I most likely would not have had that reaction.

Fortunately, I didn't go into a flashback. I took no action I would regret later. I started to think the therapy was working.

WHOP, WHOP, WHOP, WHOP, WHOP. The sound of rotor blades slice the air as the helicopter flies low overhead and then touches down nearby. The yellow smoke from the grenade tossed to mark "caution" at the LZ swirls up and in circles. The chopper blades churn the air, the tree branches, the grass, and me. Squinting against the flying road dust, I help to lower the wounded marine from the side of the Duster and into the outreached arms of other marines. They hurriedly carry him in the poncho we've been using as a field stretcher to the chopper for dust-off. They load him on the pilot's side while two other injured marines are lifted onto the chopper and laid next to him, perpendicular to the open doors on each side. Three other wounded marines step in without help.

Just as quickly as it came in, off the helicopter lifts again. The timing was precise, just enough time to get the wounded on before the helicopter became a target itself. It quickly disappears over the tops of nearby trees.

Looking up to watch the chopper depart, I feel the vibration in my hands and hear the noise of the lawn mower running in front of me. I realize a helicopter has just flown over—a U.S. Army Reserve chopper on approach to land at our local airport.

Taking several deep breaths, I stop the mower. My heart pounds so hard I think it would burst out of my chest. First kneeling on the grass, then resting on my back, I wait to recover from yet another flashback.

3

California Dreamin'

Mom and Dad, can I use the car so Tim and I can go to Huntington Beach tonight? The grunion are running!"

That morning in July 1966, Robert W. Morgan, the disc jockey on KHJ radio, called out to Los Angeles as he did every morning.

"Good Morgan Boss Angeles!" The pitch of his voice rose with excitement.

"It's seventy-six degrees in downtown LA. The time is nine-eighteen on a groovy Friday morning. Don't forget the grunion are running tonight!"

At nine that Friday evening, Tim and I sped out to catch Southern California grunion. We cruised down Huntington Boulevard, past the citrus and palm trees planted in the center divider, the windows down as we sang along with the Beach Boys, "I wish they all could be California girls."

As we approached the beach, we recognized the familiar smell of oil pumped from the noisy, black, grasshopper-like rigs that dotted the area, gently nodding up and down pumping oil. Then suddenly the smell of oil evaporated into the scent of salty air and the feel of the cool ocean breeze on our faces.

I hadn't always lived in California. I was born in Memphis, Tennessee. Mom and Dad hailed from Illinois. Dad had been stationed at Fort MacArthur at Los Angeles Harbor after the war and told Mom he wanted to return. Therefore, in 1955, when I was seven, we packed up and moved to California.

I grew up in the land of sunshine and cars. Next to the elementary school across the street from our house, an abandoned farmhouse stood on the edge of an old orange grove. It was a spook house to us kids, one of those old homes built high up off the ground to protect its foundation against flood. It seemed like a big place, maybe two stories, with lots of angles to the roof and tiny windows where someone inside could hide and watch us. None of us ever got further than a couple of steps up the porch steps before we ran down shrieking in playful fear. We chose up sides and played battle in the orange grove, picking up rotten oranges to throw at our rivals. The ammo was plentiful. We played until about four-thirty each day or until someone got hurt. Then we ran for home.

Dad was a gentle man. He trained to be a jeweler after the war, and worked at that trade until he died, but music was his love. He was a talented musician; he played clarinet and saxophone. While in Europe and later at home after the war, he had been the leader of a big band. We always had music in our family. I tried the accordion because Mom was a fan of Myron Floren of the Lawrence Welk Show. I took lessons for a few months, but I was not particularly good at it. Eventually, I ended up playing the clarinet.

At school, my life revolved around playing in the Covina High School Marching Band. We wore heavy red and white uniforms, polished white shoes, and tall white hats with gold bands and white feathers. Our band played at football games, parades, and band competitions. We were pretty good and were invited to be in the Rose Parade and different band competitions all over Southern California. We even recorded two albums.

The summer after high school turned out fun, hanging out with friends and spending time with my best friend Tim.

Tim and I never did catch a grunion. We never even saw one of the small silvery fish that come out of the water late at night to lay their eggs in the wet sand.

But we had a lot of fun in Dad's 1958 Buick Special. It withstood a lot of punishment at my hands but never gave up, and Dad never had to know. It was a solid car, a sort of sand gray with tail fins, accentuated by a chromed metal strip that started just past the back door, continued across the top of the rear fenders, and came to a peak at the rear tail light housing. It had a Dynaflow transmission, basically a one-speed transmission with $P, R, N, D,$ and L on the shift lever. I floored the throttle until the car reached about ten miles an hour, then pulled the shift lever down into low. The tires chirped out a small squeal as I accelerated to about thirty, and then I pushed the shifter back into drive and the tires squealed again.

One wet winter night, with Tim egging me on from the passenger seat, I executed spin-outs around a light pole in the Alpha Beta Market parking lot. Even in winter Southern California gets so little rain that the oil isn't washed away. When it does rain, the road surfaces are slippery. I practiced spinning the car tight on the oily, wet pavement in an open area of the parking lot a couple times. When I felt more confident, I decided to spin out around the light pole.

"Far out!" said Tim.

I gripped the steering wheel with white knuckles, as we laughed and shouted our excitement.

Six of us were cruising one Sunday evening after evening church services, and I was showing off my driving skills, again in the Alpha Beta parking lot. One of the girls in the back seat tried to throw what was left of her vanilla milk shake out through her rear side window. Unfortunately, the window was still up. The pale yellow sticky slime ran down the window, dripped over the door panel, and trickled onto the carpet. We panicked about how we were going to get it cleaned up. Somehow, we did, and Mom and Dad never found out, or at least they never said they did.

One evening in August 1965, Tim and I went shopping for a birthday gift for Tim's father, who liked to fish. Tim decided to get him a new fishing reel. It was after dark, probably around nine-thirty again, I was driving Dad's '58 Buick. We were traveling up Rowland Avenue from Citrus Avenue on the way back to my house when we decided to pull over to the side of the road and look at the fishing reel. While sitting there with the car dome light on and with our heads down intently looking at the reel, a Covina police officer stopped behind us and walked up to the driver side window.

"What are you boys doing?"

"We ain't queerin' or nothin'," I quickly responded. "We're just looking at this new fishing reel!"

After he finished laughing, he told us to go on home.

It didn't bother me that I didn't have my own car and had to drive my parents'. It was OK that it wasn't a chick magnet like a Chevrolet Corvette, a Ford Mustang, a convertible, or the "Shiny Red Super Stock Dodge" the Beach Boys sang about. I didn't mind that it wasn't gnarly. It did not make girls smile, wave, and want to talk to us. The Buick was none of those things, but neither were Tim nor I. We weren't losers, but we weren't jocks either. Neither of us was ever called a hunk. We may have been on the outside edge of hip. We were just two eighteen-year-olds, best friends since grade school, wearing button-down collar shirts, and starched jeans with a pressed crease. We were regular guys trying to grow up, have fun, and desperately wanting to learn about sex.

Holding hands with our dates and getting a kiss at the door was all either of us had experienced.

Both of my parents worked from the time I was twelve, so I was on my own after school. For the most part I was a good kid, not too mischievous, and Mom and Dad trusted me to not get in trouble. For the most part, I didn't. Other than not doing my homework, I pretty much did what I was supposed to do.

I didn't always follow all the rules, of course. When the Helm's Bakery truck drove by each afternoon, I heard its signature whistle, ran out, and bought a cream puff or cream filled donut. Boy, those were good! Mom didn't have a rule against that, but I was a bit overweight and should not have been regularly eating such things. I'm sure she would have prohibited the indulgence if she had known.

And then there was the time that I shot a hole in the living room couch. I must have been about twelve or thirteen years old. A cousin of Mom's was visiting California from Illinois and stayed with us for a few days. He had purchased a Ruger, a single-action .22-caliber revolver. He showed it to Dad one evening as I stood by and watched. I was excited about looking at the pistol. "This was bitchin'," I thought, but I didn't say it aloud.

"Neato," I voiced.

The pistol looked just like the ones cowboys used in the movies. It had a long, dark-colored barrel with a cylinder that spun when a hand pulled against it quickly. It featured brown-wood pistol grips on the handles. It clearly ranked as the neatest thing I had ever seen. They put it back in its box and placed it on the top shelf of a kitchen cabinet where I wouldn't be able to get to it.

The next day after school, I climbed up on the counter and got the box down. I had to see and touch again the smooth, steel barrel and the rough etching on the grips. I stood in the kitchen at the doorway to the living room. The tan-and-brown fabric couch with wood side panels was about two feet away from me.

To fire a single action revolver, you have to pull back the hammer until it cocks and then pull the trigger. I don't know what I was thinking when I loaded the cylinders. I remember spinning the wheel just like the cowboys did in the movies. That means I had to have pulled the hammer back. I waved the pistol and—bang!

It had gone off. I stood with the gun in my hand and a hole in the wood side of Mom's couch. I was going to be in big trouble.

"What a spaz!" I thought.

I knew I had to clean up, and fast. I cleaned the gun the way Mom's cousin had shown Dad. I returned the pistol to its box, and set the whole package back on the shelf, right where Dad had left it.

Next, I had to fix the couch. I retrieved wood putty from the garage.. Fortunately, it appeared very similar in color to the light blond wood panel on the couch.

It was a good thing a .22-caliber bullet is small, about three-sixteenths of an inch in diameter, so I filled the hole with putty, gave it a light sanding, and put everything away.

I never said anything about it, and nothing was ever said to me.

Dad was never taught to hunt and never owned a gun. His mother died when he was three years old, and his father when he was eight. His oldest sister, who was about twenty at that time, raised him and his two siblings. Mom's father and brothers hunted most of their lives, so she grew up having guns in the home. I was given a BB gun for Christmas one year. It was a pump rifle, proving difficult to work up enough pressure to fire the BBs very far. I shot at my plastic toy soldiers, apricots on the tree, and, once in a while, birds.

When I was fourteen, my Great Uncle Earl, my mother's uncle, gave me a rifle. Uncle Earl and Aunt Dea were the only family we had in Covina, and we visited them regularly. Uncle Earl was a hunter who went out every year hunting for venison. He showed Dad and me pictures taken on hunts. He mounted a couple of prized antlers and a deer head in his den. He kept an old rifle standing in a corner of the room, near the door. It was his first gun, given to him when he was a young boy in Illinois. During one visit, I offered to clean the rifle and refinish the wood stock. Uncle Earl agreed. It took me two or three weeks to complete the cleaning and refinishing. I carefully disassembled all the parts, cleaned, and oiled them with the correct gun oil that Dad helped me buy at a hardware store. I decided to stain the wood stock a red cherry color rather than the usual oiled wood color. I sanded and rubbed and sanded and rubbed. Finally, the stock was ready for the stain and a final coat of high gloss spar varnish. To me, it was beautiful.

That weekend when we visited Uncle Earl and Aunt Dea, I presented him with his new rifle. He complimented me on all my hard work and fine workmanship.

"Do you want it?" he asked.

I guess he had already cleared it with my folks, because when he asked, I looked at them, and they both nodded their approval. I quickly accepted.

I suppose he probably wanted to hand it down to family since he didn't have a son to pass it on to. I was glad to get it and glad I had put so much effort into refinishing the stock. I was about seventeen when Tim, another friend Gary, and I drove out to the desert near Twentynine Palms to shoot at some tin cans and sagebrush. That was the only time it has been fired since Uncle Earl gave it to me. It now sits on a shelf in my closet. Someday I'll give it to my son.

FROM AS FAR BACK AS I CAN remember, I always liked airplanes. As a kid, I built plastic and balsa wood models and imagined I was flying them. When I was a senior in high school, I decided that I wanted to be a pilot. My parents, despite their payday-to-payday income, indulged me and arranged for me to take flying lessons at Brackett Field, the local airport, located over the hill in Pomona.

My first lesson was an introductory flight. It took about forty-five minutes and included some classroom instruction and some flight time. The classroom instruction covered what makes a plane fly, the components of an aircraft, and primary instruments in the aircraft. My instructor, Sonny, was about five-foot-four and balding. He wore a brown leather jacket, a white long sleeve shirt, dark slacks, and shined dress shoes. When we walked to the airplane, a PA-28, which is a Piper Cherokee 140, Sonny pointed out and explained each of the aircraft control surfaces. As he did that, he was also performing the pre-flight safety check.

Sonny told me to get in the left seat, the primary pilot's seat, also known as the *PIC* for *Pilot in Command.* We went over some information in the cockpit, and then he yelled out the open door for anyone who could hear, "Clear prop!"

"This is so bitchin'," I thought to myself.

Then, with a turn of the key, the engine came to life. The propeller in front of me was spinning and making the plane rock slightly as the thrust pushed against the tail surface. Sonny picked up the microphone and talked to the control tower, getting taxi information, wind direction, and speed. We taxied into position at the hold line at the end of the runway, and Sonny used the radio to contact flight control for permission to take off.

"PA, Whiskey Two-Three, you're cleared for takeoff. Continue straight out and turn left at the tanks."

"Roger, Brackett Control, PA Whiskey Two-Three cleared for straight out takeoff and turn left at the tanks," repeated Sonny.

Then to me he said, "Put your left hand on the control yoke and your right hand on the throttle."

I did as he instructed. Then he pressed on my right hand, pushing the throttle all the way to its stop. The little Cherokee 140 roared to life and started to roll toward the other end of the runway. With his right hand loosely on the control yoke on his side, he told me to gently pull back on the yoke when the airspeed indicator reached sixty-five miles per hour.

"Not too much — gently," he said.

As I pulled back, the nose of the aircraft began to come up off the ground. Then I could hear a quieting as the main gear tires left the runway. The plane seemed to be lighter, not that it weighed less, but so it was more controllable and took less effort to move the rudders, ailerons, and elevator.

Climbing to about one-thousand feet, Sonny gently turned the yoke to the left while easily pushing on the left rudder.

"We're over the tanks," he said.

The tanks were several large oil storage tanks that were about two miles away from the airport. They made a good reference point, because they were easy to see from the air when approaching or departing the airport.

We flew around for a little while as he demonstrated: S-turns, approach and departure, stall turns, and slow flight, which is controlling the plane at a speed just above its stall speed, the slowest speed at which it can safely fly.

"Where do you live?" Sonny asked.

"In Covina."

He pulled and turned on the yoke and pressed the rudders to turn the plane around and head for my home in Covina. He asked if I could find my house, and I did. He then turned the plane steeply into what is known as a 720 About a Point, that is, making two complete 360-degree circles, so that the tip of the left wing pointed at a spot on the ground. In this case it pointed at my home as we circled it from above.

That was my first flight lesson, and I loved it from the start. The whole time we were flying, I actually held on the yoke and flew the plane. After that I took a lesson about once a month and before long had my first solo flight.

When I look back, I understand how naïve I was in high school and junior college. I didn't have any real plans for life. My parents continued to pay for my flying lessons at Brackett Field, and I wanted to be a pilot; but I didn't have anything planned out.

"THE BEAT GOES ON." I carried my transistor radio with me and sang along with Sonny and Cher, the Beach Boys, and the Monkees. I was just a kid, and life was copacetic.

But there were other songs on the radio that didn't make much sense to me. What did Bob Dylan mean, "Blowin' in the Wind?" In addition, I sure didn't get all the gloom in Barry McGuire's "Eve of Destruction."

However, one popular song in 1966 I understood. For five weeks, Staff Sgt. Barry Sadler's "Ballad of the Green Beret" ranked number one on the charts.

4

The Evening News

O ne American soldier was killed today on Tan Son Nhat
Air Force Base in Vietnam."

Walter Cronkite announced casualties every evening on
the six o'clock news. We talked about the war in my high school
civics class, but I didn't think much about it—that is until the
draft loomed over all our plans and changed our lives.

When I registered with the selective service on my eighteenth
birthday in 1965, I knew guys were being called up to service.
By June of 1967, when I had completed my first year at the local
junior college, the war's effect on me was becoming clearer. For
a while, my local draft board had been granting deferments for
those enrolled in college. However, as time went on and the need
for fresh recruits increased, the government tightened up on
deferments. I knew I would be drafted.

I considered my options. I heard of a friend's older brother
going to Canada to avoid the draft. For me, that was not a
consideration. I couldn't leave my country, and I couldn't
understand anyone who would. To me the choice was clear: two
years or four. I had heard it was possible to volunteer to be drafted,
and that by volunteering I could request when I wanted to be

called. Military enlistments required a four-year commitment while the draft imposed two years' active duty and two years in the reserves—unless stationed in a combat zone, which meant that reserve time would be served as inactive reserve.

All four military branches were involved in Vietnam. The air force had air bases located all over that country. The navy kept ships off shore and small riverboats inland. The army and marines, of course, were on the ground. It didn't matter what branch of service I entered; I would most likely go to Vietnam.

I had heard guys talking at school about each of the branches— army, navy, air force, or marines—to pursue a particular training and job duty while in the service. As it turned out, they got the training, but after that, they went where the service wanted them, whether it involved the training they got or not.

My best friend, Tim, had tested for the air force and scored in the ninety-ninth percentile in mechanical aptitude. He wanted to do something that would allow him to be on a flight crew, including service as an aircraft or helicopter mechanic. When he was at the recruiting office, Tim was told to put down three preferences. For the first, he put aircraft mechanic. For the second, he put helicopter mechanic. He saw, on the list of air force occupations, the term "munitions specialist." For the third, he checked that box. He was gone by July first, off to attend a munitions specialist school.

It seemed rather silly to be sent off to serve four years for his last choice. I thought, "Why should I do four years of something I don't want to do, when I could do only two years of something I don't want to do?"

I volunteered for the draft. It was June, 1967. I wrote a letter to the Selective Service Office local board in Pasadena, California, telling the board I wanted the summer after the current semester in junior college to be with my friends and that in the near future, perhaps in September, they could call me for the draft.

Two weeks later I received a draft notice telling me to report to the Los Angeles Examination and Induction Station, 1033 S. Broadway, Los Angeles, at eight in the morning, September 4, 1967.

"Wow, that was quick," I thought.

They didn't waste any time at the draft board. The letter gave me a level of certainty. I was nervous, yet at the same time, it was calming to know what would happen and when.

I tried to make the most out of the rest of my summer. About the same time in June that I wrote to volunteer for the draft, I met a pretty girl named Bonnie. She worked at the May Co. in the Eastland Mall in Covina. I did a lot of shopping at the May Co. for a couple weeks before I got the courage to ask her out on a date. We spent a lot of time together those remaining months.

MOM WOKE ME SHORTLY AFTER SIX O'CLOCK the morning of September 4. I smelled bacon and heard it crackling in the skillet as I dressed. When I got to the kitchen, Mom was already fully dressed, her hair styled and makeup on. I don't know when she got up, but, as usual, she was fully dressed and ready for her day. That morning she wore a dress with a colorful apron that tied behind her neck and in back around her waist.

She had made bacon and eggs with fried potatoes and toast. She knew it was my favorite breakfast. She fried the eggs in bacon grease, cut the potatoes in large bite size pieces, and added diced onion, bell pepper, salt and pepper, and other spices. The potatoes had browned—crispy edges, but tender inside, probably dusted in flour before frying to give them the crisp edge. The onion and peppers became translucent in the large cast iron skillet, all fried with bacon grease and a little extra Crisco from the can always found in Mom's kitchen.

Usually Mom was talkative in the morning, asking me questions about what I had planned for the day or telling Dad and me what she had planned. Some days she hummed a tune to herself. But that morning she was conspicuously quiet, concentrating on the meal. No hummed tune and no conversation. It was as if she were alone and needed to concentrate on what she was doing, forcing out all other thoughts.

Packing for my trip proved easy because the draft notice said to just show up with what I was wearing along with my toothbrush, shaving cream, and razor. The week before, our next-door neighbor had come over with a gift for me, a shaving bag. He said that he'd had one when he was in the army, and he'd found it useful. He hoped that I would find it useful as well. It was a tan, imitation leather bag with a zipper across the middle. It was just large enough to hold my basic hygiene items: a bar of soap in a two-piece plastic container; shaver with twist handle that would hold and flex a double-edged razor; Babasol aerosol menthol foam shaving cream; tooth brush; a tube of Colgate toothpaste; and an extra pair of skivvies rolled tight.

At seven-fifteen, Dad and I got in the Buick. Mom, now with the tears she had been holding back, said good-bye. Dad backed out of the driveway, and we headed down the road toward the LA Examination and Induction Station for my eight o'clock appointment.

We tried to make small talk about the weather and how light the traffic was at that time of the morning, but that was not what was actually on our minds. It was only a thirty-minute trip, but with the uncomfortable silence, it seemed longer. We sat in silence and stared at the road ahead. Left turn onto Hollenbeck Avenue down to Citrus Boulevard, then right onto the Interstate 10 into Los Angeles.

The Selective Service building stood as a tall, gray edifice, three stories, set back from the curb thirty feet with a concrete sidewalk in front. Uniformly spaced on either side, two large square holes in the concrete opened up for trees—maples, about ten- to twelve-feet tall with branches full of green leaves spread out and beyond the planting holes. The touch of green showed brilliantly against that gray structure, probably a Los Angeles beautification requirement. To me that morning they looked out of place, as if intentionally concealing the truth inside.

Four heavy columns fronted the building with a pedestal base on the concrete rising to a matching podium at the top of the building. A thick, coarse screen, perhaps some sort of security screen, covered tall and narrow glass windows on the front of the building. The effect of that tall imposing gray structure was ominous and out of place next to the lower, smaller buildings on the street. It made me feel that something important or frightening would happen when I went inside.

As we pulled up in front of the building, Dad gave me some advice: "Do what your drill sergeants tell you to do and don't volunteer for anything…or at least be careful what you volunteer for," he paused, "because when I was in the army, getting a person to volunteer would usually be a trick for some kind of work detail or at least something I didn't want to do."

He gave a short simple laugh, perhaps at a memory briefly passing through his thoughts. Then he turned to face me, looking through his glasses and with his pleasant smile, he said, "You're my son and only child. I love you and will miss you."

He reached over and gave my left shoulder a firm squeeze. These were words I had not often heard my father say.

5

Marching to a Cadence

I walked through the doors to a long day of standing in line, filling out papers, being tested, prodded and probed, wearing only my socks, shoes, underwear, and t-shirt.

Shots. So many shots. They had a contraption like a chrome pistol with two short barrels. It had hoses hanging from it that went to large bottles hanging from a rack. There were two of these, one on the left, one on the right, each operated by a nurse. When I was next in line, a nurse directed, "Relax your arms and stand still."

Then just as she finished speaking—*bzzt*—they shot me in each arm.

"Step forward."

Bzzt. They shot me again with another double-barreled shot pistol. Two more paces forward and *bzzt,* I was shot again. The shots were pressure injected; they didn't use a needle; they felt like any other shot, but the noise was memorable. A kid three places ahead of me in line jerked his arm when they tried to give him his shots. It cut two deep slices in his arm. They bandaged him up and scolded him for not doing what he was told. He took the shots again. At the end of the day, he was on a bus with the rest of us.

I hoped to get into the army flight program and told the medical examiners so. Maybe I should have kept my mouth shut. Maybe they didn't like being told anything by an inductee. When the examiners checked my vision, they told me it was only twenty–twenty-five, not good enough for flight training. That was bullshit. I already had a student pilot license and a flight physical that showed I had twenty–twenty vision. When I tried to tell the doctor (or maybe he wasn't a doctor, but a frustrated assistant mad because he wanted to be a doctor), he snarled, "You're wrong. Move on!"

That was my first encounter with the harsh reality of the army. I was frustrated at not being able to make my situation known to someone who cared. I didn't try too hard; I was scared and intimidated by the induction processing. I felt that was it. There was nothing I could do, so it was just move on, and welcome to the army.

The induction process took all day. It was late afternoon, and the sun was setting when we moved outside to fill four waiting school buses. We didn't know where we were going. I had heard that most guys drafted on the West Coast were sent for training in the east, and vice versa. That did not turn out to be right, and I had no idea where we were headed when I got on that bus.

The buses cast long shadows stretching out across the sidewalk and up onto the building. I looked out the bus window and saw a marine sergeant and an army sergeant standing on the sidewalk talking. Then the marine sergeant pointed to the bus in front of the one in which I was sitting. We knew that whole bus was going to be drafted into the Marine Corps. The bus erupted with guys shouting and trying to climb out the windows. Military police officers with their nightsticks appeared and hit the hands and bodies that were trying to get out of the bus. That bus went to

Camp Pendleton; the other three buses, including mine, went to the army installation at Fort Ord, California.

When the buses pulled out and on to the freeway, the noise and conversation inside turned quiet. We all were physically tired and emotionally exhausted. The trip to Fort Ord probably took a little more than six hours. It was close to midnight when we arrived. It had been dark inside the bus as we drove, but when the bus stopped, the interior lights came on. Most of us had been asleep, so the stop and sudden lights startled us awake.

When the bus doors opened, a tall, slender black man entered the bus. He was wearing shiny black boots that came about ten inches up the shins of his legs. The toes of his boots reflected the light as if there were mirrors on them. He was wearing an all green uniform with matching hat. The uniform was heavily starched and pressed with creases that looked sharp enough to cut a rope. The hat had a brim that was perfectly flat all the way around, like the one Smokey the Bear wears. A brown leather strap circled the base of the hat and made a strap that went under the edge of his chin.

His first words were shouts, telling us he was going to count to twenty, and if we weren't all off the bus and standing at attention in a formation parallel to the bus with rows four deep, we would have to do it again.

He stood there in the doorway and started counting. The first kid up bumped him trying to get out of the bus.

"Whoa, whoa, whoa! What the hell do you think you're doing touching me?" he shouted.

"Get back on this bus and in your seat, you piece of shit, and if you ever touch me again, you maggot, I'll stuff this size-twelve boot of mine up your ass so far you won't be able to shit for a month!"

This time he got off the bus, stood next to the door, and

started counting. When ten of us were off the bus, he shouted: "Twenty—Everybody back on the bus! You lowly, stupid ass, lazy sacks of shit had better learn how to follow orders and be quick about it. Now do it again."

This went on two more times before he finally let us all get off and try to stand at attention in a reasonable formation.

"Welcome to the United States Army. You're at Fort Ord."

Then he told the kid standing at the front of the first row to lead the formation over to the building with all the lights on. It was a cool night with a slight ocean breeze, but I was sweating nervously. As we walked, he yelled some more obscenities at us and sang out a marching cadence: "Yo lefty, right, a left...Lefty, right, a left."

It wasn't until the next day that we learned to repeat and sing back the cadences.

Inside the building, despite the late hour, we were given a sack lunch that contained an apple, milk, along with a peanut butter and jelly sandwich. We sat on folding chairs and ate for what seemed only seconds before he ordered us to stand up, throw what remained of our meal in a trash can, and stand in line to go into the next room.

In that room, long rows of white folding tables were all set up and spaced exactly the same distance apart. Folding chairs were uniformly spaced at each table as well, with a sharpened pencil in front of each, the point of the pencil pointing at the exact center of the chair. We were told to sit down and, even though it was late, fill out more papers. After all that was finished, we went outside and, accompanied by more cursing and insults, marched to an old wooden barrack that was temporary housing for that one night. Actually, our marching was probably more like walking in a group than it was marching in formation. I don't know what time it was when we finally got to go to bed.

I had barely closed my eyes when I was startled by the sudden loud blaring sound of a bugle being played over a speaker and the drill sergeant standing in the doorway of the barrack yelling, "Get up, you panty waists. You ain't gonna get any beauty rest in my barrack. Stand at attention at the front of your bunk!"

It wasn't even light outside; the lights had to be turned on. It would continue this way for the next eight weeks.

"I am Staff Sergeant Henley. I am your drill instructor."

"If it is absolutely necessary for you to speak to me, you will address me as Drill Sergeant, or Drill Sergeant Henley. When I talk to you, you will answer me by saying, 'Yes, Drill Sergeant.' Do not call me 'sir'; I am not an officer. That would be a waste of my talent and abilities. I will be your drill instructor for your time here at Fort Ord. I am not your mother! I *will* be your counselor, spiritual advisor, and your worst nightmare. Is that understood?"

After a brief pause, "I can't hear you...."

Again, there was a nervous pause, which was almost deafening. Then, he shouted louder still, "I still can't hear you!"

It took several tries before we caught on, and all yelled back in a scattered, not-yet-unison, response, "Yes, Drill Sergeant!"

After that, we marched to a mess hall for breakfast. That first full day was used to get haircuts, uniforms, boots, shoes, socks, bedding, towels, and assorted army necessities, and more tests! We took eight categories of tests, assessing our aptitude for job training that the army determined would suit us best.

6

Going to the Beach

L ater that afternoon, we were marched to what would be our barracks for the rest of basic training, a fairly new, two-story concrete structure with a central front and back entrance and stairwell. It was designed to house four platoons, one whole company, one on the left side, and one on the right side of both the first and second level. We were now the Second Platoon, Company D, II, BCT. BCT stood for Basic Combat Training. More than fifty of us in our platoon were housed on the second floor on the right. There were eight of these barrack buildings in the training area. Each barrack housed a company in a different phase of training, spaced one or two weeks apart, a continuous supply of trained replacements. Entering our barracks, I saw a row of bunks lined up on each side of the room. Because my name was close to the beginning of the alphabet, I was assigned the second bunk on the right. In front of each bunk was a wooden trunk, a footlocker painted flat olive-drab, the army's favorite color. At the foot of each bed, about two feet away against the wall stood a tall metal locker. The center area, between the two rows of bunks, measured about ten feet wide with a single black six-inch-wide line extending from the threshold to the far wall.

We were instructed on the rules of army barracks life, how to place every piece of our clothing and equipment in the footlocker and wall locker. Socks and underwear had to be folded a particular way with stitching in an exact alignment. Toothbrush, shaving razor, and soap each had its specific location and direction of placement in the footlocker. There were rules for hanging our clothes in the wall locker. Every footlocker in the barrack was to look exactly the same as every other footlocker. Each wall locker must look exactly like every other wall locker.

There would be an inspection! Every day, either with us standing at attention next to our footlocker or while we were out of the barracks at training, inspections surveyed the entire building and our individual bunk areas. Any discrepancy meant a demerit and some kind of punishment.

Punishment usually consisted of extra physical training (PT). Sometimes it meant extra PT for the whole platoon. That carried a lot of peer pressure. Extra PT usually consisted of running one or two extra laps around the barrack, which was probably close to a quarter mile total. Individual PT would always include at least twenty or thirty push-ups. Every trainee at some time received a demerit for something being out of place. I came to believe it was a requirement of the basic training experience. If extra PT was not assigned, spit-shining the centerline was.

DI Henley barked at us, "Without exception, nor tolerance, do not touch, step on, scratch, mar, or in any way deface or cause to be defaced, *my* center line!"

The line had to be kept shining at all times with the highest luster possible by shining it with spit and boot polish. I remember being down on my knees and sometimes on my stomach, with a can of black boot polish and a white cotton rag using my saliva to shine a section of that stripe. First, I wiped my rag into the can and scooped out some black polish. I spread it onto the floor line in a circular motion, being careful not to get any polish beyond the edge of the line. The polish had to be rubbed in until it became smooth, then I spit onto the floor where I had just applied the fresh polish. Using the clean, soft-cotton rag, I buffed it out to the highest possible luster. This is the same process used on shoes and the toe and heel of boots for a spit shine.

At each fall out, we made a coordinated and panicked effort to avoid touching that line as we exited the barrack, usually at a full run, and DI was always there to observe that we did so. Nearly every day, two or three of us were called out for some variety of assault on the line and given the responsibility of spit shining the line after dinner mess.

There was no meaning to it. It was done to add an extra level of stress to our training. I imagine the DIs had a big laugh at the end of each training graduation, comparing each class' experiences with the line.

I didn't think so back then, but in retrospect, I understand the DIs had a tough assignment. No matter how early we were awakened and roused out of bed for training, the DI was always already standing there looking strack, in perfect order, in his perfectly starched and creased uniform, spit-shined boots and stiff brim hat, shouting out insults, obscenities, and orders. Nor did his day end until after ours was over. In addition, I know the army always had paperwork to be done on top of it all.

Fort Ord is on the Monterey Peninsula. In those days, the entire base seemed to be covered with sand. We marched in sand, did pushups in sand, and ran in sand. As anyone who has ever walked on the beach knows, when you walk in sand, it pushes away from your feet, offers less resistance to push off from. It requires twice the effort to move in. Sand became just another drudgery of basic training.

OUTSIDE THE MESS HALL ENTRANCE, a sand pit had two horizontal ladders, or monkey bars. Before each meal, we lined up in front of the bars. DI or one of his cadres was also standing at the bars. As we stepped forward to the horizontal ladder, we stated our name, rank, and military ID number. Then DI asked a question, or told us to recite one of the six numbered statements of the Uniform Military Code of Conduct. After answering, we had to do ten push-ups, get up on the horizontal ladder, do two pull-ups, walk the ladder, and do two more pull-ups on the opposite end, before dropping off to go inside the mess hall, just to get in line again to get a tray full of food and all the cold milk we could drink.

OF COURSE, EVERY TIME WE MARCHED, we marched to a cadence. Some cadences were inspiring, and some were quite demoralizing. DI called out a cadence and we repeated it. He sang, "Left...left...left, right, left...gi'me yo left...gi'me yo left."

He sang a cadence, "Jody's got your girl at home."

Then we repeated, "Jody's got your girl at home."

In turn, the DI said, "They'll be gone when you get home."

And we repeated, "They'll be gone when you get home."

"Am I right or wrong?"

"You're right." we obediently responded.

"Am I right or wrong?"

"You're right."

Each time the word left or right was used in a phrase that was the foot I was stepping down with. At times, DI would change "Jody's got your girl," to "Jody's got your car," or anything else he could think of. By the end of the first week of basic training, Jody had possession of everything that was good, everything I had I had to leave at home! Jody was a dirty, no-good, rotten snake in the grass.

In another cadence, DI said, "Your momma was home when you left."

We responded, "You're right."

The DI continued, "Your daddy was home when you left."

"You're right."

"Momma was home...daddy was home...everyone home when you left."

"You're right."

"Break it on down."

"1, 2, 3, 4, 1,2...3,4."

There were other cadences like, "I want to be an airborne ranger."

"I want to drop down from the sky."

"Hooah...Hooah."

On the east end of Fort Ord, the sand stretched inland for several miles. I know because when we went on a twenty-mile march, there was still sand everywhere. I'm sure we didn't actually march out ten miles and then turn back. What we likely did was march in zigzags and circles until we returned back to the barrack after twenty miles. One thing I know for sure: there was sand everywhere along the route, with scattered bushes and evergreen trees growing in the sand. As I said, Fort Ord is located in the Monterey Peninsula, and that means the beautiful and serene towns of Monterey and Carmel were only a few miles away, about ten minutes by car. However, we never saw the historic, scenic parts of the Monterey Peninsula, but we saw a lot of sand.

Every platoon has a Dud. A *Dud* is the name given to a person who seems to have trouble doing nearly everything. They are not always problem people, but just someone the DI picks out for harassment more than anyone else. Our Dud was chosen because he made some mistakes the first day, putting things in the wrong space and alignment in his footlocker.

Dud had trouble making military corners on his bed. When making your bed in the army, there is, like everything else, a specific way to do it. There is a bottom sheet tucked in at the head and foot end of the mattress. The excess sheet is then pulled tightly around and down, to create an exact forty-five-degree angle at each corner of the bed, and then tucked in under the side of the mattress. On top of that is, of course, the top sheet and blanket, with the top tip of the sheet folded down precisely over the top edge of the blanket and again tucked in to make a forty-five-degree angle at the bottom two corners. A second blanket is also placed on the bed, and it is folded in exactly four folds and draped at the foot of the bed with equal portions hanging over each side. When all this is completed, if the sheets are properly tucked, the mattress will tend to be ever so slightly curled up at the edges, causing a tight stretch across the bedding. The true test was when the DI flipped a quarter on the center of the bed, and it bounced back up. If it did not bounce, he turned the whole bunk upside down and told the hapless trainee he had only five minutes to make it up correctly with military corners and a perfection that would pass the bounce test. After taking this much effort to make a bed, it wasn't long before I, and most everyone else, learned to get into bed, sleep without moving, and get out in the morning without having made much disturbance in the bunk. Dud never figured that out.

One day we were at the rifle range on the beach where large sand dunes rose up nearly a hundred feet above the shooting platform. All shooting was toward targets at the base of the dunes, with the Pacific Ocean on the far side. We were ordered to go to the prone position, which is lying on our stomachs. The M14 has a flash suppressor on the end of the barrel that is about three-inches long. It has three prongs connected together with a ring at the end. One prong is on top and the other two are at an equal angle and space apart to the bottom, causing the muzzle flash to be separated, and causing more down force on the barrel after recoil. I don't know for sure what happened, but I suspect that when Dud dropped to the ground, he must have allowed the end of the barrel to go into the sand. Dud was at the position on my left. DI gave the command to commence firing.

When I heard the *ka-boom*, I looked to my left and started laughing. The flash suppressor of Dud's rifle had flared open like the end of an exploded cigar in a Marx Brothers' movie. "Oh shit! DI's going to kill him," I thought

"Cease fire, cease fire!" screamed DI, as he ran to Dud's position. He then hit him on the head with the firing range safety sign. Fortunately, we always had to wear a steel helmet.

Man, what an ass chewing! DI threatened Dud with court martial for being stupid, destroying government property, and for embarrassment to him and our entire platoon. I felt bad for Dud, but secretly glad it wasn't me because it easily could have been. I suppose that it could have been dangerous—no one knew where the bullet went after it hit the sand and then the end of the flash suppressor. I'm pretty sure that it would not have hurt anyone behind the end of the barrel. I don't know if he was too scared to say anything or if he didn't know there was an obstruction in the end of his weapon, but when he pulled the trigger, that round hit the obstruction when exiting the barrel. Everyone within hearing distance knew, there would be hell to pay for that one.

That night in the barrack, we all laughed. Some of us tried to console him. It's still funny after all these years. I'm laughing out loud as I write this story. I remember the end of that M14, with the three blades of the flash suppressor completely blown open and all three tines flared out about ninety degrees to their side.

Much of our time was spent in the classroom. After rising at 0500, followed by hours of PT, staying awake listening to the instructor drone on was difficult. Our DI had a solution to help us stay awake in class. I know it worked because he used it on me more than once. As soon as he saw my head drop, he shouted my name, "Blaylock!"

I jerked my head up.

"Go to the back of the classroom and stand at attention for the rest of the class period."

By the end of the class, as many as eight trainees would be standing at attention along the back wall of the room.

7

You're in the Army Now!

The obstacle course was probably only about a mile long. When we reached the third or fourth week of basic training, we ran it two or three times each week. The obstacles included walking or running a rail, getting over a net about twenty feet high, climbing a wooden tower with horizontal bars twenty-five to thirty-feet high, crawling through a tube, jumping a hurdle, and climbing over the dreaded wall. The wall is a simple, flat wooden structure, six feet high by about twelve feet wide, supported on each end by large timbers to keep it from falling over when I ran into it. I never could get over the wall. Each day when I'd start the course, I'd feel my anxiety mount, my pulse rise, and my sweat running. I'd tell myself I had just started the course and should not be that sweaty. As we ran the course, some of the guys taunted me, "The wall is coming up."

Others tried to encourage me, "You can make it today!"

It was a splendid opportunity for Drill Instructor Henley to badger and curse at me. He had a remarkable talent for allowing things to spew forth from his mouth, and no matter what words he used, they sounded vile. They were the undeniable truth according to him and the U.S. Army.

Day after day I ran up to the wall, stumbled, pulled, grunted, groaned, and tried to get over that blasted wooden structure. Even without the seventy-pound pack on my back I could not climb over that stupid wall. A couple of times, I was able to sneak around the wall without being seen. The DI caught on, and after running around it one day, I ran right into him waiting on the other side.

After I completed my fifty push-ups, I had to go back around to the front of the wall and attempt to go over again. The DI yelled, threatened, and even instructed me as to how to get over. One time he actually pushed me over. Each day, after several attempts, he would finally shake his head in disgust and tell me, "OK, Blaylock, go catch up with the rest of the platoon." One day, probably in about the seventh week of our eight-week training, I tried yet again several times to get over that damn wall. Each time I succeeded only in running into the wall, not over it. DI Henley, after yelling his usual obscenities, even tried to help me. He did not help physically, by pushing me, but he helped with his own distinctive way of encouragement.

"Swing your leg up over the goddamn wall and hook your ankle over the top edge, so you can pull yourself up and over!"

Each time I swung my leg up; I fell to the ground on my back.

"Come on Blaylock, damn it, get your fat ass over that wall."

Of course, I wasn't the only one in my platoon who couldn't climb over the wall. There were two other guys who couldn't get over it either. But as far as I was concerned, it was only me.

Finally, DI Henley called everyone back to the wall to do it again, and this time to help, and if necessary, push those of us who needed help over the wall.

We learned to help each other not just over the wall, but whenever someone needed help, including Dud, so we could fight together as a whole unit. By that point in our training, DI's goal was to teach us to work as a team, a whole fighting unit is better than one man short. When we started basic training, we were individual recruits. We didn't know each other and only made relationships according to where home was. There is a semblance of connection to home in a group of strangers when you know someone grew up anywhere near your hometown.

Basic training was tough both physically and mentally. There was a lot to learn and to do just so that we could go on to Advanced Individual Training (AIT), our next training assignment. In only eight weeks, a short two months, DI taught us to work together as a single unit. It would be an exceedingly long time before I would see this as a positive experience, but I did think to myself, "When I weighed in at the Induction Center, I was 189; now at graduation my weight is 160. What the hell, I lost nearly thirty pounds and added muscle. I am looking good!"

While in basic training, I wrote letters to my girlfriend Bonnie every chance I could. As trainees we could only make phone calls on Sundays, so every Sunday I called Bonnie and my parents.

FAMILY AND FRIENDS WERE INVITED TO ATTEND a graduation parade and ceremony when we completed basic training. My parents drove up from Covina and brought Bonnie with them to Fort Ord. The parade and ceremony consisted of our marching up and down parade grounds about the size of a football field, followed by a few speeches by the training brigade commander who was a colonel, then followed by a lieutenant general, colonel, a major, and two captains, as well as a couple of our training DIs. It was DI Henley's speech that meant the most to me because it was he that I had worked so hard to please. After the ceremony, we had leave to go off base for the rest of the day; we did not have to report back to barracks until 2200 hours.

In spite of my inability to get over that damn wall, I guess I must have done OK because DI Sergeant Henley recommended me for promotion to E-2, and it was granted. I would be able to sew a chevron on the sleeves of my uniforms. Dad was proud when I told them all after the ceremony.

Dad drove the four of us in the 1966 Buick Wildcat into Monterey. We walked along looking and talking before we settled on a restaurant on Cannery Row for a celebration dinner. We sat next to a view window that looked out on the Monterey Peninsula. The waiter wore a black tuxedo jacket with a white shirt and carried a white napkin over his left arm whenever he came out from the kitchen. I was impressed that he did not write anything down but was able to serve us each exactly what we had ordered. The restaurant smelled of fish, but what I remember most was the bread and butter. The bread was crunchy on the crust and soft, very soft, on the inside. The crust wasn't hard or chewy like sourdough, just crisp or brittle; it made a crackle sound when it was torn apart, and flakes of crust scattered all over the white tablecloth. The inside was so soft with all the little air bubbles from when it was baked that it would crush down to almost nothing when pressed between my fingers. The butter was so smooth and creamy when spread across the bread. Somehow, it reminded me of the special potatoes Mom had fried for me the morning I left home.

I WAS SENT TO FORT SILL, OKLAHOMA, for my advanced training in artillery. I trained there from early November until late January, with a one-week leave for Christmas. I learned how to operate 105-mm and 155-mm Howitzer cannons to become an artillery gunner.

While stationed at Fort Sill, I was called to report to the base band director, a major, to audition. After a short interview and audition, he told me that I should return to my training platoon and not wait for his call.

On Thanksgiving Day, I called Bonnie and asked her to marry me. She said yes and instantly started making plans. In 1967, males had to be twenty-one-years old to be fully emancipated. What that meant was that my parents would have to sign a paper giving me permission to get married. I came home for two weeks on Christmas leave, and we were married on December 30, 1967. After a brief two-day honeymoon, I returned to Fort Sill to finish my training. Fully trained by January, I got orders to attend a two-day jungle school and M16 rifle training. Further orders quickly followed to report to Fort Lewis, Washington, on January 20, 1968, for deployment to Vietnam.

My parents petitioned the army not send me to Vietnam because they said I was a sole-surviving son. They contacted their congressman asking him to support their request that I not be sent to Vietnam.

When I arrived at Fort Lewis, my orders were put on hold pending a decision on my parents' request. While waiting to hear, I continued to process with all the other guys to go to Vietnam. The army issued me new jungle fatigues and boots after I turned in my uniform and fatigues. These new fatigues fit loosely and featured large pockets with button-down flaps on both shirts and pants. The new jungle boots had canvas sides and ventilation holes that supposedly were better for my feet, allowing them to air-dry more quickly.

I did not tell my parents, but I wanted to go to war. I think my desire to go to Vietnam started sometime during boot camp. I hadn't talked to anyone about my feelings. Perhaps I was afraid of being labeled a warmonger if I mentioned it. I figured that if I told anyone, I'd probably get a bunch of flack for it, so I kept it to myself. I had heard guys say things about how they wanted to go kill some gooks, but that was not what I was feeling. I just felt this was what we were all doing, and I needed to go ahead and do my part. I thought I could do something for my country. It gave me patriotic pride. I felt embarrassed that my parents were trying to keep me from going to Vietnam.

Their petition created a delay in my ship out, so I was temporarily assigned to a desk job at a headquarters company. I was at Fort Lewis an additional four weeks before the army made its decision. They told my parents that the law did not apply to an only child or son; it was intended for surviving brothers.

"Pack your stuff Blaylock… you're movin' out!"

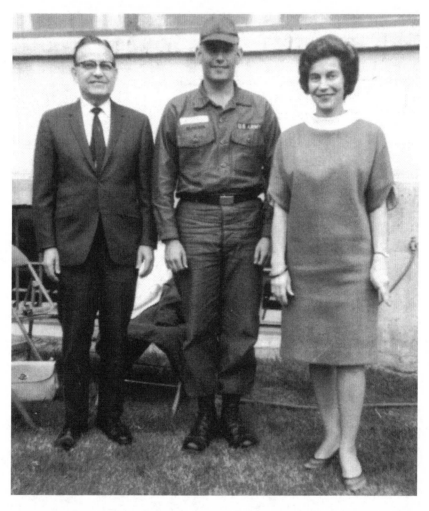

Bill Blaylock, center, with his mom and dad at U.S. Army basic training graduation at Fort Ord, near Monterey, California

8

A Cloudy, Overcast Day

At the Seattle Tacoma airport, I walked in line from the flat, olive-drab army bus out to the shiny white and red Boeing 707, chartered from Western Airlines. A giant red W branded the tail, and a long red line continued down the side of the plane. We stood in formation at parade rest, and then, row-by-row, we were called to attention and marched single file to the waiting aircraft. I remember multiple airplanes parked on the ramp waiting for us to board. Once again, just as when I'd left Los Angeles, it was late afternoon. The sun in the western sky cast long shadows on the ground. I climbed the flight stairs where a sergeant directed us as we filed in to occupy each spot, row-by-row and seat-by-seat. I took a center seat on the right side of the plane. The sun shone through the windows on my left and onto the floor of the center aisle.

It was March, the temperature mild, but ever so slightly cool, with remnants of a morning rainstorm and an overcast of high clouds. It was the kind of chill that makes you shiver just a bit to disguise the uneasy nerves. I was feeling anxious about all the standing and waiting. It was something I always did in the army but never got used to. Maybe it was because I was about to go to Vietnam, or maybe it was just because. Because of what, I don't know. There was a low buzz coming from a few guys attempting to talk to their seat partner. Flight attendants moved up and down the aisle, offering magazines and reminding us to buckle our seat belts.

The silence…it was deafening. The door of the airplane was pulled shut and locked, like the shutting of the door on a bank vault. It did not actually make much of a sound, just the sliding of the door bottom rubbing across the edge of the carpeted floor at the threshold. It was a sudden and deliberate sound that seemed to take away my breath and seal my fate. The silence was everywhere and lasted a long time. I began to hear the whine of the jet engines starting. There was a slight shake of the plane as the ground tug began to push the plane into position for taxi.

"Bye, Bonnie," I thought. "Bye, Mom and Dad."

We roared down the runway, passed the runway lights, and then saw airport buildings blur by faster and faster. The plane vibrated under my seat on the floor, under my thick-soled black, shiny boots with the green canvas tops, up my legs and into the pit of my stomach. But the rumbling didn't stop there; it continued up through my chest, out my arms and into my fingertips that gripped the seat armrest with white knuckles. Although I loved flying, and jet flight was not new to me, this time was different. I had never felt like this before. Hearing the thundering, powerful sound of the jet engines just as the plane started to rotate up excited me.

"Yahoo, let's go get 'em!" someone yelled.

The whole inside of the plane came alive with excited, anxious talk. We were going to be warriors! That yell was a yell of relief, releasing the tension each of us felt but didn't admit. The plane filled with high-strung chatter.

What was ahead? What would happen when we landed? We did not have weapons—how would we fight? It turned out, of course, that there was no small-arms fire or artillery incoming at the airbase in Cam Ranh Bay when we landed, but I did not know that until I got there.

I have tried to remember details about the flight to Vietnam, but the only thing I know for sure is that it was dark when we landed in Japan to refuel, and it was morning when we arrived in Vietnam. When I calculate the flight time from Seattle Tacoma Airport to Cam Ranh Bay, Vietnam, including the refueling delay in Japan, we must have been en route about twenty-two hours: Seattle to Japan, 5,000 miles; Japan to Cam Ranh Bay, 2,300 miles; 7,300 miles divided by a flight speed of 350 mph is just under twenty-two hours. Not long after takeoff we were served a warm prepared meal. Some hours later, not yet asleep, but trying to rest with my head back in the seat and my eyes closed, I heard the crew announce over the loud speaker, "Buckle your seat belts; we will be landing in Japan to refuel."

The aircraft doors didn't open. I watched through the windows as the fuel truck operator completed his job. "Buckle up for takeoff." This time there was little enthusiasm; we were tired and apprehensive, not knowing what lay ahead. The morning sun was bright, shining a warm yellow-orange light through the windows as the stewardesses passed out boxed breakfasts.

9

'Goood Mornin' Vietnaaam'

G ood morning, gentlemen," the airline captain announced. "The time here in Cam Ranh Bay is 1035 hours. The temperature is eighty-eight degrees with a relative humidity of ninety-two percent. You guys take care."

Looking out the window, I saw a base so large the only things visible were pavement, hangars, and cargo buildings, blurred by the heat waves rising from the open tarmac. I was relieved that there did not seem to be a need for having a rifle and ammo before getting off the airplane.

The doors of the aircraft opened. Hot, humid air rushed in. The smell of that air burned into my mind; it has remained there ever since. The humid atmosphere seemed to surround me, like a wet, warm blanket wrapped around my body. It filled my nostrils as if a poisonous gas were trying to overtake me. But it was not a gas, not a poisonous one, not one that would take me down instantly. It was the smell of Vietnam. It smelled of sweat, of the vegetation of the jungle, of mildew, of pain, of fear, of death. It is impossible to explain—but the smell in the air singed the fine hair of my nostrils as it made its way to my lungs and burned itself into my memory.

A lieutenant who had come aboard near the front of the plane ordered, "Move out!"

A portable stairway was pushed up to the plane, and the lieutenant stood next to the door as we passed by to exit. "Turn right at the bottom of the stairs and follow the sergeant."

We walked rather than marched. It felt strange to exit with no formation, no lining up, and no cadence. We just walked, not in a straight line, but as a group, staggered and undefined. We walked to an open hangar about a quarter mile away. The sudden change in military formality did not feel right. To me, it should have been more controlled, rather than relaxed. Inside the hangar, clerks sat at tables, six to eight of them. Some of the clerks ranked as private first class and others as specialist fourth class. They were wearing baggy jungle fatigues; some had pockets buttoned and others did not. They looked out of uniform. Some smoked while they worked. There were one-gallon cans scattered about, retrieved from the mess hall, painted red and half filled with sand, to use as butt cans. Behind each table stood a sign with a series of letters: A–C, D–G, and on through the alphabet.

We got into lines according to the letters of our last names and waited our turn to talk to one of the clerks. It was a long wait in the sun before I got inside far enough to be in the shade of the hangar roof. It must have taken an hour for me to get to the front of the line. They had a list of our names and military occupation specialties. When I checked in, the clerk I talked to looked tired and bored. I asked how late they stayed to process in new troops. He told me that they have continuous shifts, twenty-four-hour processing. I took directions to find my duffle bag from the pile that had been tossed on the ramp just outside the hangar and then waited until my name was called, at which time I would get my orders.

"It'll be a few hours, so if you're hungry, there's an open canteen next door."

I retrieved my duffle bag and walked to the canteen. They had a breakfast line and a dinner line. I could take whatever I wanted. I had never experienced anything so relaxed in the army: just get what you want, sit down, eat, and then make room for someone else. Back at the hangar, I found an open spot on the floor in the area where I was told to wait. Several more hours went by before I was called, given papers, and told to report to the hangar next door to catch a plane to Da Nang.

This time the wait was only a couple of hours before boarding. It was a bumpy ride in the C-130, sitting in sling seats that hung on the inside walls of the aircraft, with palletized cargo strapped down to the floor. The C-130 was a four-engine turbo-prop cargo plane with a fold-down, rear-cargo ramp for vehicles to drive onto. Through porthole windows, I could see lush green trees of the jungle as we flew north to Da Nang. Other than in movies, I'd never seen a jungle before. It was thick with trees and plants growing so close together that I was unable to tell where one separated from the other.

We arrived at Da Nang Air Base Fifteenth Aerial Port Squadron, and I reported to the office at the rear of another large, open hangar.

"Make yourself comfortable until you hear your name. It'll be a while," advised the clerk.

I hoped this wait wouldn't be as long as the first. Looking around, I spotted a small patch of unoccupied floor next to a wall and near the large front opening of the hangar. Until then, I had been so focused on myself I had not seen any farther than my own personal space. But, as I made my way to what would become my spot for several hours, it became clear to me that this place was full of GIs, all waiting for their names to be called. It was a huge hangar, large enough to park at least two large planes inside. Instead of planes, it was filled with GIs, maybe three hundred or more, all sitting, standing, or lying on the floor, talking to one another, trying to fill the time and to understand what was going on. It was a rolling sea of olive-drab fatigues and duffle bags. The skin of many colors, black, brown, and white could be seen at the collars and sleeves of the fatigue uniforms. We were all there, all the races of America. We were young, mostly eighteen- to twenty-years old. We were, for the most part, as clean as can be expected after spending so many hours on the floor of aircraft hangars; after all, we were incoming replacements. Some were tired, some anxious, some pissed-off, and some, I'm sure, scared.

I was tired and frustrated more than anything else. I wanted to just get to it. The noise level in the hangar rose and fell continuously with occasional outbursts of laughter from one or another group where a joke had been told.

It was there, sitting in my spot waiting to be called, that I met Leonard Bruski. When I found that vacant spot on the hangar floor that I called my spot, Leonard was already sitting down next to it. I would spend the rest of my year in Vietnam with him. I would come to know him well as a combat buddy and as a friend. He was a solid, muscular young man of nineteen years with sandy brown and curly hair only visible when he removed his hat because of his military haircut. We introduced ourselves, and I asked where he was from.

"Alpena, Michigan. Way up north. You can see Canada across the bay from it."

In his speech, I detected a slight accent I had never heard before, not strange or funny, just different. We spent the time making small talk and taking short catnaps to alleviate boredom. He seemed to be a good guy and easy to talk to; I liked him. He had worked at a factory in Alpena, and would probably go back to his job when he got out of the army. He had a high school sweetheart, Julie. He took out his wallet and showed me her picture, and I showed him a picture of Bonnie. We made several trips to the twenty-four-hour mess hall, more from boredom than hunger. It seemed we spent days right there in the hangar, but it was actually just the rest of that day, all night, and several hours the next morning.

Months later, toward the end of our tour, he would write in a photo album that I bought from a vendor by the road, "That's when it all started."

Finally, about twenty names were called, including Leonard's and mine. We were told to get on the deuce-and-a-half, a versatile utility truck used for practically everything in the military. In this case, it was used as a taxi. The truck was waiting to take us to our next flight, after which we'd report to headquarters battery. The truck took us about a mile away and stopped beside an aircraft that I had never seen before. It had two turbo-prop engines and what looked like tiny jet engines hanging from pylons under each wing. To me, they looked as if they were just recently bolted on, as if somebody decided to add them at the last minute. However, they matched the weathered paint scheme, so I knew they belonged there. The plane was dirty with scratches on the fuselage and wings, and it had a tall tail that swept up from the top of the fuselage. The fold-down, rear-loading ramp looked as if it needed repair.

As we walked up the loading ramp, I asked the loadmaster, "What is this thing?"

"It's a C-123," he snapped. "Find a seat!"

Just like the C-130, the C-123 had sling webbing on the inside for seating and for strapping pallets to the floor. There was no cargo on this flight, just us twenty soldiers with our duffle bags. The plane taxied out to the runway and revved up the engines for takeoff. As we started to roll, I heard a loud, high-pitched whine from those tiny jet engines, and just then the aircraft rotated skyward at an amazing rate of ascent. In all the flying I had done, I had never climbed at such a steep rate. It wasn't long before the plane leveled off for cruise. The noise level inside the plane was loud. I got up, walked over to the loadmaster, and asked him where we were going.

"Dong Ha," was the response.

"Where's that?"

"You'll find out soon enough. Sit down, we'll be landing soon."

I looked out one of the four windows on my side of the plane. I could see we were flying much lower than before, probably no more than two-thousand feet above the ground. This time I could see and make out the definition of the individual trees of the jungle below.

"We'll be landing in just a few minutes. Grab your bag and be ready to get off when the cargo ramp is fully down."

As he finished talking, he pulled a lever near where he was standing, and the loading ramp started to open.

Just then the plane made a steep bank left and dropped altitude quickly to the runway. There was a loud bang as the landing gear hit hard against the steel-landing grid on the ground. The pilot suddenly seemed to be in a hurry. Time had sped up in urgency I didn't understand. Something must be wrong. The cargo ramp was going down, and the loadmaster screamed at us,

"Get out! Get out!"

The plane was still rolling down the runway, the cargo ramp almost dragging on the ground, when the loadmaster started throwing out duffle bags and pushing us out.

"Get out! We're taking fire. Get out!"

"What do you mean we're taking fire?" I asked.

"They're shooting at us, stupid. Get out!"

Holding my duffle bag and running out the ass end of the moving plane, I found a ditch on the side of the runway to jump into and covered my head with my hands and duffle bag. It took mere seconds to unload the plane, and it never came to a complete stop. The pilot pushed the throttle to full thrust. I looked up to see it almost instantly airborne, flying away to safety.

Slumping there in the ditch, I remembered my earlier fear of not having a rifle to fight back with in case of attack. "What the hell's going on here?" I wondered. "I'm going to die right here before I even get a chance to fight back!"

I could hear the explosion of mortars hitting nearby. I later learned they were not so close. I also heard small arms fire in the distance on the other side of the airport. The enemy didn't have accomplished aiming capabilities and would re-direct their mortars until they reached their target. With time, I was able to distinguish between what was either distant or what was imminent danger.

As I waited with my head down and hands covering it, all I saw was the red of the Vietnam soil. In fact, the red covered everything: the equipment, vehicles, buildings, and uniforms. Everything that had been olive-drab was now red.

A siren sounded briefly. I could see people starting to come out of the ditches and holes in the ground. I later learned that those holes in the ground were below-ground bunkers. Leonard and I found each other and went to the building labeled "headquarters." We gave our papers to the clerk. Leonard asked him, "Does this happen often?"

The clerk said casually, "Four or five times a week, but usually only when there's a plane on the ramp."

By now more guys were coming into the office. Pointing to Leonard, me, and one other guy, the clerk said we were being assigned to First Battalion, Forty-Fourth Artillery, One Hundred-Eighth Artillery Group. I figured that meant that I would be on a Howitzer, probably a 105 mm or 155 mm, like the ones I had been trained on at Fort Sill.

"Headquarters Battery is at Camp Carroll," said the clerk.

Each battalion had a headquarters battery and from two to seven batteries, labeled A, B, and so on; most commonly, there were four batteries per battalion. A Headquarters Battery resembles a large company that has several sales divisions. The Headquarters Battery is where the boss is, the battalion commander.

Camp J.J. Carroll, named after a marine major, was located in I Corps, which I later found out was pronounced, "Eye Corps," not "One Corps." Vietnam was divided into four military areas of operation. Each had a Roman-numeral designation, I thru IV. The corps, or sectors, started at the Vietnamese Demilitarized Zone (DMZ) and continued south through the entire country. The DMZ was a dividing line between North and South Vietnam.

The third guy assigned with us put out his hand. "Hi, my name's Dennis, Dennis Ramsey. Yu'n boys c'n call me Cefus."

Cefus, Leonard, and I would spend the next twelve months together, brothers for eternity.

10

The Journey Continues

Leonard, Cefus, and I rode the sixteen dusty, bouncing miles from Dong Ha to Camp J.J. Carroll in an open deuce-and-a-half with six other guys. Our truck took the middle position of a convoy of nine vehicles, including supply trucks, jeeps, and two Quad 50s, one in the front and one at the rear of the convoy. The Quad 50s, a two-and-a-half-ton truck with low sideboards, protected us with their four, .50-caliber, power-assisted machine guns, mounted on a turret and manned with a crew of four: one gunner, two loaders, and a driver.

Trees and jungle brush lined both sides of the rough road, which climbed over hilly terrain. After fifteen miles of potholes and small craters, the wooden bench seat in the truck bed reminded me of the swats I got with a wood paddle when I was in high school. The dean of boys had caught me and another kid leaving campus to smoke a cigarette. Even though I was wearing jeans, the paddling left a red mark on my butt. The hard, wooden slats of the truck seat would certainly make a similar red mark. With all the bouncing, only the truck's side-stakes kept us from falling out. I did not see any other people or vehicles moving on the roadway. Red dust swirled up from the tires onto and into everything, even my nose, ears, and mouth. It was gritty in texture, like the fine sand I sometimes found in the hamburgers, hotdogs, and fries from the boardwalk vendors at Huntington Beach.

We were traveling on a Vietnamese road, Highway 9, which I would travel almost every week during my one-year tour of duty. Although regularly graded by American bulldozers, it was a poor dirt road. It had seen frequent battles and was scarred by powerful munitions and enemy land mines. It was the responsibility of the morning road-mine sweep teams to find and detonate land mines and clear the roads for daily commerce.

We traveled the road at a steady speed, maybe twenty-five mph for about half an hour. I was feeling tense with nervous idleness and had just lit my third or fourth cigarette when I heard *pop, pop, pop*, the sound of rifle fire ahead of the convoy. Those of us riding in the truck dropped to the floor to take cover. The drivers of all the vehicles immediately opened the throttles and drove as fast as they could go without hitting the vehicle in front. They drove fifty- or sixty mph, staying in the tire tracks of the vehicle in front to avoid hitting a land mine.

In a situation like that, the drivers want to get away as fast as possible. Peeking up over the sides and back of the truck, I saw marines from some of the jeeps and trucks starting to return fire, shooting into the surrounding trees. The two Quad 50s opened up with a great roar, spraying hundreds of rounds of blazing hot .50-caliber lead into the trees and brush around us. Then, suddenly, the firing stopped, and the convoy slowed back to its original pace. We got up off the floor of the truck and continued along as if nothing had happened.

"What the hell was that?" asked Dennis.

We, the three Cherries, looked around and at each other.

"What did you see?"

"Nothin' but the floor of this truck. What did you see?"

"Just trees and bushes going by."

No one else on the truck seemed to be excited about it, so we shut up. I didn't exactly feel scared, but rather pumped up with adrenaline.

We traveled about ten more minutes before we started up a fairly steep road. A whistling sound broke the not-so-peaceful quiet: *ssssooouu!* Again, explosions and gunfire rang out.

Guys yelled, "Incoming!"

The convoy stopped. Artillery and rockets fell all over our location. We abandoned the vehicles, quickly following the other soldiers, jumping into ditches that lined each side of the road. The explosions were larger, louder, and closer this time. They were also more frequent.

"Mortars," someone yelled.

"Rockets," yelled another.

I don't think they really knew, but it didn't matter. "Either one would kill me!" I thought. I could tell the explosions were much closer than the ones on the runway at Dong Ha. I kept my head down and prayed, "Lord, please let me live through this unharmed. Don't let one land on me."

Leonard found himself in a ditch next to a marine who was a short timer. He had about thirty days left in the country. They talked a bit. When Len told him he had just arrived in the country two days ago, the marine sold Len his K-bar, a marine-issue knife, for a dollar. He told Len, "If I still had that much time to do in this shit hole, I'd kill myself!"

The words scared Len and haunted him the whole time he was in Vietnam and for years after. Then just as quickly as it had started, the attack was over. We got back in our vehicles and continued up the road to the base camp, just a half mile away.

I soon learned that all might be peaceful with no sense of impending danger when, instantly, fighting could erupt. Other times, I might be warned by my sixth sense, what I call a sick sense. I soon developed a sense that told me when something was wrong. I noted the absence of villagers on the road or something different, but I was unable to put my finger on exactly what. At other times, all felt peaceful with no sense of impending danger. Then my sick sense failed me, and shots would ring out. But this day everything was new. Not yet at my assigned destination, and I'd already survived three attacks.

The convoy arrived at a large open area where the vehicles joined others parked in several widely spaced rows. Cefus, Leonard, and I walked a hundred yards to a reddish-tan building that had sandbags stacked around it, from the ground to the roof. A sign over the entrance read, Headquarters Battery, First Battalion, Forty-Fourth Artillery.

Inside, a specialist fourth class, sitting behind a desk, greeted us. "Are you guys the new replacements? Give me your papers!"

He looked at the papers for a while, made notes on others lying on his desk, and said we were assigned to "First of the Forty-Forth, "C" Battery, First Platoon, Second Squad." He told us to take a seat while he called our squad leader, so we seated ourselves in the folding chairs set against the wall behind us.

Soon a young black man walked in. "Hi, I'm Cuba C. Wright, your new squad leader."

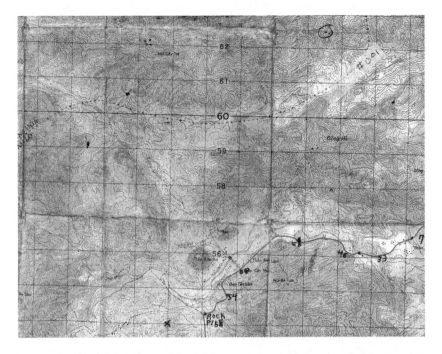

Leonard brought home this folded map of Vietnam. Rockpile, OP Ben, is marked with an *X* at the bottom left along the 54th Parallel, Highway 9, and Song Cam Lo River. The DMZ is at the 60th Parallel. Khe Sanh, not indicated on the map, is about eleven miles by air, east- south east of Camp Rockpile.

11

The Duster

Our squad leader had a big smile with white teeth, but when I think of meeting Cuba, I think first of the hat he took off as he walked into the room. He wore it everywhere. He took it off only when inside or to put on his steel helmet. It had once been olive-green but was now dusty-tan with a dark sweat ring around the base of the hatband. It wasn't a regular army-type ball cap, but a pliable, flimsy, fully brimmed hat that no longer held its shape. I had never seen one of those hats before, but I soon saw that nearly everyone had one; before long, I had one too. Cuba was about five-foot-nine and wore a specialist-four rank pin on his shirt lapel. He would come to be a valued friend and the person on whom I would most rely. I wish we could have maintained our friendship back home after the war.

We told him our names, and he shook our hands.

"Did you say Cuba, like the country?" I asked.

"Yeah, just like the country." When he spoke, I detected a slight New York, or possibly New England accent. I never asked and he never said how or why he got that name.

"Come on with me to our hooch, and you can meet Soo."

We walked about a quarter mile to the hooch, a structure that looked similar to the headquarters building, also with sand bags stacked two-deep up around the sides and top. Wooden pallets were spread out on the front side of the hooch, giving the appearance of a porch, where a folding, web-laced patio chair and a long couch with broken-down, dirty cushions welcomed us.

"Hey Cuba, where'd that couch come from?" I asked.

"I don't know. It's always been here!"

As we approached, I noticed a tracked vehicle parked close by. More sand bags were stacked around its parking area. Then about thirty feet farther out, rolled barbed wire and several strands of taut, barbed wire fashioned a fence line. Beyond that, perhaps another twenty yards, the landscape had been cleared with Agent Orange and graded clear of brush and trees so that no one or no thing could approach without being openly exposed.

Camp Carroll sat on top of a hill, the highest in the area, giving us a fair view of the area and any enemy movement. All the vegetation was green—dark, dark green. The fighting had obviously disturbed some areas, but even there, most anything that had not been destroyed by fire or explosion was still green. The jungle recovers quickly.

Once inside we met Spc. 4 Soo. He was a tall guy about six-foot-three with short, black, curly hair. Soo told us he was from San Francisco and that he was the driver.

"He's the driver of what?" I wondered, but didn't ask.

Inside, the hooch was dark, with a single low-watt light bulb in a socket hanging near the middle of the room. For light, there were candles and you could always use the flame from your "Zippo" lighter, or your army issue flashlight with its red lens, less visible than white light. The hooch was about fifteen-feet wide and ten-feet deep with a low ceiling of about no more than six-feet high. I thought it odd that the ceiling was so low because other hooches were higher than ours. Soo, had to stoop over when he walked inside. They had placed five cots around the room near the walls, just enough for one crew, indicating to me that it would be only us five staying there together. One cot was occupied and another must be Cuba's, since it had scattered paper and a pen lying on it as if it had been put down in a hurry. I realized he must have been writing a letter when the clerk called him to come get us.

The walls were plywood with large timbers supporting the corners. Four more timbers extended from floor to ceiling about every five feet through the middle of the hooch. Their spacing allowed room for a single square wood table with two wood chairs directly under the light. This completed the décor. Cuba had us put our duffle bags down on a cot, which had a greenish-brown, wool blanket stamped "U.S. ARMY," folded and placed at one end.

"Come on outside, and I'll show you the Duster."

"Isn't this a Howitzer battery?" I asked.

"Naw, that's too safe. We've got this Duster."

The M42-A1, commonly called the Duster or sometimes a track (a generic word to describe any vehicle that ran on tracks rather than wheels with tires), was a self-propelled, anti-aircraft weapon. It took its nickname from all the dust it churned up from the dirt roads when it traveled. It could run at speeds up to around forty-five mph, quick for a tracked vehicle weighing nearly twenty-one tons. It was powered by a Lycoming, gasoline fuel-injected, air-cooled five-hundred horsepower engine. Being a tracked vehicle, the Duster didn't need roads. I would soon learn that we could drive over small trees, ditches, and even through water up to three-feet deep. The problem with deep water was the Duster usually got stuck in the mud at the bottom. We tried to avoid water without a sandy or rocky bottom. The Duster had two 40-mm guns that could fire 240 rounds per minute. The ammunition rounds would travel about three miles. Every round was a tracer, so it was compelling to watch and follow the rounds flying to their target. Each projectile weighed about two pounds and was sent out the barrel with a muzzle velocity of 2,870 feet per second.

Our company commander wanted each crew to name their dusters something that started with the letter C for C Battery. The five of us came up with Cobweb Crusader, and I painted a big spider web on the shield that separated the two guns. We were C121.

"Blaylock, since you're a PFC, you'll be the gunner. Leonard and Dennis, you guys are the cannoneers."

As PFC, I was a higher rank than Len and Dennis.

Within a few weeks, Cuba filed papers for my promotion to E-4, and Len and Dennis to (E-3) private first class.

The crew consisted of a sergeant, a gunner, two cannoneers, (one for each of the two 40-mm guns) and a driver. The sergeant, gunner, and driver all had helmets with communication speakers plugged in with a long, twisted, coiled cord. The Duster could carry six personnel. A second seat in the front hatch could accommodate a lieutenant or observer if one ever came along. But most always it was the five of us.

Refueling was a pain in the ass. I had to crank the hand pump every time we went down to base camp for fuel. The four of us, Soo, Cefus, Len, and I took turns cranking the pump from fifty-five-gallon-barrels of gas through that damn manual pump. The Duster's fuel tank held 140 gallons. Each time we got fuel, we used two full barrels plus part of a third, which meant we couldn't have had more than thirty gallons left in the fuel tank. That's a lot of hand pumping!

The Duster carried all we needed. In addition to the 350-plus rounds of 40-mm ammo and each of our individual M16s, it stored extra cases of C-rations, water, and blankets for the occasional overnight missions. If necessary, we could attach a small trailer behind the Duster to carry extra supplies, like sand bags, shovels, ammo, and C-rations.

The Duster first deployed in Vietnam in 1966. The M42-A1 was actually an upgrade from the M42. A1 came from a change of engine, which added fuel injection in 1956. About 3,700 were manufactured, and they were supplied to some NATO countries. They took a key role in Korean air defense. With very little North Vietnam aircraft, they became effective against ground forces. With their heavy firepower, the Dusters were capable as security perimeter defense and for mobile convoy escort missions as well as morning mine sweep defense and protection. The Duster was phased out in December 1971, replaced with newer, rapid-fire, self-propelled weapons.

The sergeant-squad leader and the gunner sat down in the turret with only heads and shoulders exposed above the turret rim. However, the cannoneers had to stand up in the turret area to fire and had to lean outside the turret area to retrieve ammo stored along the side. The driver came up on deck to assist the cannoneers to retrieve ammo if he was able.

Because the Duster was fast and could fire while moving, it was high on the response call-out list, and was feared by the Viet Cong (VC) and North Vietnamese Regular Army (NVA). They nicknamed it "Fire Dragon."

Cuba took us up, down, and around the Duster, explaining everything and how it worked.

For the rest of the day, we learned how to operate, maintain, and take care of our new, (at least to us) equipment. Cuba got clearance to practice fire. For the next two days the five of us practiced running from inside the hooch to our positions on the Duster. We would fire several rounds at a target; usually a tree on a hill located across the valley from our hooch on the perimeter of Camp J.J. Carroll. Those first couple of days of training were filled with running out to the track, firing several rounds, then cleaning the guns. Each morning after breakfast at the mess hall, we went back to the hooch and practiced our run, fire, and clean process two or three times. Then we took a break to write letters home and play gin rummy, which began a seemingly never ending routine of cards, cigarettes, letters, and, sometimes, a reading of my Gideon's New Testament. It was the way I spent much of the rest of the year.

"We're the perimeter guard, the first defense; if anyone comes through the perimeter line, they'll meet us first," warned Cuba.

Cuba wanted to impress on us that ours was a quick-response piece of equipment and that quick action was required for us to be able to both defend our perimeter and save the lives of ground troops when called out to their location. I realized this later, when, after the riflemen, we were the first to return fire when sent out to respond to a call for assistance. We had both the ability to supply rapid, heavy firepower and to travel off road.

Cuba had a daily meeting at headquarters where he was briefed on the day's activity and the next morning's assignments. When he returned from his meeting on the second day, he told us that the next morning we would be assigned to escort a convoy along with another Duster and some marine grunts. The convoy would be from Camp Carroll to Dong Ha and back.

Someone asked, "What do we do?"

"Just ride along until they shoot at us, and then we'll shoot back," Cuba said, with a sort of snicker in his voice.

That's all that was said, and we continued the card game. A few more cigarettes and a couple more gin rummy games completed the evening. It was usually Len, Dennis, Cuba, and I in the card game. Soo seldom played.

It was difficult to sleep that night. At 0600, I awoke to the playing of reveille by a bugle on the camp public address system.

After breakfast, at about 0700, Soo had started and was warming up the Duster. By 0715, we were rolling into position for the convoy, and by 0730 we were moving out. We passed through the gate guarded by marines and down the steep, winding road toward Highway 9.

I was tense as I continuously looked and listened while riding along the road. My gunner's helmet had a microphone and speakers that allowed Cuba and me to communicate. In the open turret of the Duster, I sat on the left side and Cuba sat on the right with the two guns and Dennis and Len in the middle, between us. I guess that I must have been talking too much, or talking to myself, because I heard Cuba ask a question.

"You OK over there? You seem nervous."

"Yeah, I guess I'm all right, aren't you nervous?"

Cuba just laughed and told me to relax and enjoy the ride until something happened. When or if it did, I would know what to do, he assured me. I felt like a candy ass, and he was my big brother trying to protect me. It was embarrassing letting my nervousness be so obvious. After what seemed to be only a few minutes of riding along, I looked at my watch, the one that Mom and Dad gave me before leaving home to report to Fort Lewis; it had been nearly half an hour since I talked to Cuba.

"OK," I said to myself, "you've got to relax."

I started to observe my surroundings. The road was lined on both sides with deep ditches. Trees of the jungle vegetation had been cut back and away from the edge of the road. Partially destroyed and burned out-buildings dotted the landscape. I started to relax. There wasn't any threat, and then I thought to myself, "This isn't so bad." Although monotony abounded, little did I know that it would not always be this way.

We made it all the way to Dong Ha, loaded supplies on the trucks, and returned to Camp Carroll without firing a shot.

Convoys traveled continuously throughout the entire country during daylight hours; it was too dangerous to attempt travel at night. They carried supplies and troops to wherever they were needed. They traveled from major airports and seaports to base camps, then to smaller, more remote camps.

From there field operations could go to the remote camps to get their supplies. They carried food, ammo, fuel, people, mail, and everything else needed to conduct a war properly.

Each convoy needed security to help protect it from attack. When a convoy was attacked, one Duster and a truckload of marines would engage the enemy while the rest of the convoy sped ahead, accompanied by another truckload of marines and the other Duster. I didn't learn this routine until several days later when we finally took enemy fire. We also called artillery and air support to our position. Later, our split convoy would meet up farther down the road, if possible. When encountered by a larger enemy force, the convoy would continue without waiting to reunite with those of us who stayed and fought, and called for backup and air support. Backup usually meant calling an artillery strike onto the suspected enemy location. That usually solved the problem. However, sometimes a situation required the aid of airborne firepower, like army Huey Helicopter Gun Ships, air force F-4 Phantoms, or A-1 Sky Raiders.

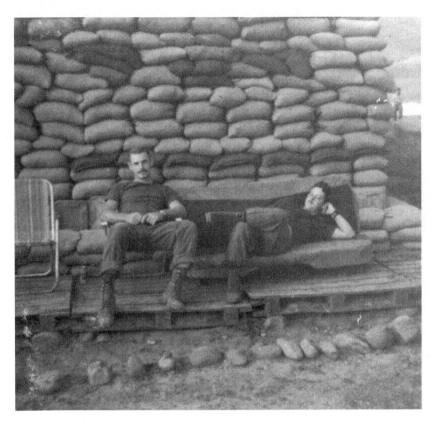

Leonard and Shorty relaxing in front of the bunker at Camp J.J. Carroll

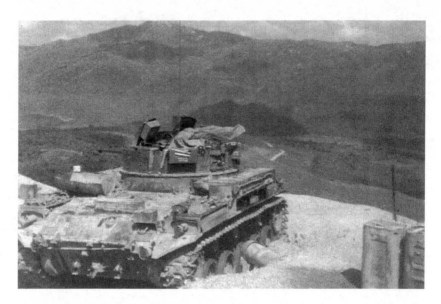

The M42-A1 "Duster" with its twin 40-mm guns was known to the North Vietnamese Army as the "Fire Dragon."

12

My New Home

Six weeks after my arrival in country, April 16, 1968, we moved from Camp J.J. Carroll to a place called the Rockpile. Camp Rockpile was located between Camp J.J. Carroll to the east and Khe Sanh to the west in the Quang Tri province on Highway 9. Camp Rockpile earned its name from its location at the base of what looked like a pile of rock, rising seven hundred feet to tower over the surrounding country.

Two observation points (OP) overlooked the Camp: OP Able and OP Ben. We were on OP Ben, about a mile and a half away and on top of a hill overlooking Camp Rockpile. Our battery rotated on an unscheduled routine, between the Rockpile and Camp J.J. Carroll.

Marines occupied OP Ben, usually with a squad, sometimes two, with a single, Jeep-mounted 106-mm Recoilless rifle. They had encircled the perimeter with coiled barbed-wire fencing, three-feet deep and about five-feet high. Marine sniper teams used OP Ben as a base from which to operate for a month or more. During our stay, several sniper teams left from and returned to our hill.

When we arrived in mid-April, the marines had already carved a space for the track to park and had dug out a place where we would build our bunker.

Building our bunker started as an exercise in futility. None of us knew anything about constructing a building, let alone building a bunker designed to withstand a lot of weapons fire without collapsing on its occupants. Proper construction required significant design and sturdy materials. Most bunkers in our part of Vietnam seemed to be constructed of large timbers, plywood, corrugated metal, and sandbags, lots and lots and lots of sandbags. Our ignorance about how to do it notwithstanding, we got to work.

Before we started building the bunker proper, we filled sandbags, ammo cans, and boxes for days. We stretched out some canvas tarps between a small trailer loaded with the building supplies and the ground. We used it as our temporary day- and night-time shelter. We created so many sandbags that we began to like the idea of sleeping under that tarp. We filled fifty or more 40-mm ammo cans, which were about twelve-inches square and maybe twenty-inches tall. We also filled about fifty wood ammo boxes and sandbags, which we piled everywhere along with some lumber and plywood.

Shoveling dirt was tough, and digging the piss tube wasn't an easy task either. A piss tube is a plastic or metal tube partially buried in the ground. From bottom to top, sand follows a layer of small rock, overlain by a larger rock, then a covering of dirt. The design allows the tube to protrude above the ground about two feet. Urine seeping into the tube can filter into the soil.

We stacked ammo cans five-high in the middle of the bunker and put a two-by-four-inch board vertically on each side to stabilize the cans. Then we placed boards across, from the side to the central ammo can column and layered plywood on top of that. Soo was on top catching and placing while we made a sand-bag brigade tossing them up to him. Soo had placed about ten sandbags or more on what was to be the roof of our new bunker and home when he yelled out, "Oh, shit!"

We watched as the whole thing started to collapse and then fell down with him on top, riding the sandbags down as if he were surfing a wave around our wonderfully conceived center support column. Amazingly, when it was over, Soo was left standing, unhurt in the middle of all the dirt and dust. The cloud of dust must have blown out forty feet. We stood there looking at each other, covered with the filthy red-clay dust and dirt, and then started laughing.

The next day a lieutenant came up to tell us what to do and how to build a bunker that would not only stand on its own, but would be able to withstand enemy weapons fire well enough to protect those of us living in it. Why we didn't get an engineer up to help and instruct us sooner, I'll never know.

We did build our bunker, and we lived in it. We entered through a canvas flap doorway. Two bunks were on the right and three straight across on the opposite side. I had the top bunk on the right. They were comfortable bunks made of wood ammo boxes nailed to two-by-four-inch boards. Two folded woolen army blankets made up the mattress, and I used a rolled-up towel for my pillow. I wrote a letter to my parents on May 14, 1968, and told them we were almost finished with construction and that "our bunker leaks."

We hung mosquito nets over our bunks, but they only kept out small, flying insects. The bigger crawling things weren't slowed down at all. Cuba and Soo had done an admirable job of instructing us about the dangers of bugs in Vietnam. Some are extremely poisonous. Before getting into our bunks, we had to check them for critters, like scorpions and centipedes. Centipedes grew to a pretty large size, eight to ten inches or more, and delivered a much more venomous sting than that of a scorpion. Scorpion stings would just make you sick and run a high fever for a few hours. A centipede sting would most likely put you down for an entire day with pain and fever. The scorpions I saw were usually two, or at most, three inches long. I never knew anyone who had been bitten or stung, but I believed what Cuba and Soo told me. I usually slept with my boots on so I could blouse my pant legs inside them to prevent bugs, snakes, and rats from crawling up my legs while I was asleep. I tucked the bottom couple of inches of the pant legs into the tops of the boots before tying the top laces. If I didn't blouse my pants, I would at least tie off the pants leg at the bottom with a boot lace.

Poisonous snakes were prevalent in Vietnam. The most poisonous and common snake in our area was the Bamboo Viper. The Viper was a tree snake that had earned the nickname of the Two-Step Viper. Legend held that, if bit, you had time to take only two steps before falling dead. I don't think there is actually anything that deadly, but it made for a good story to keep troops on their guard.

The rats—the great big rats—I hated them. Nearly every night I woke to one walking up my leg. I would kick it off, hear it hit or fall against something, and go back to sleep. Rats ran everywhere in Vietnam, and they were enormous. Rats were in their usual environmental places. They preferred dark, secluded places, like my bunker. They made nests in the thick, tall grass, in wood, and rock piles. Although they are primarily nocturnal, occasionally they would run in open areas and across the road during the day when we were on a mine sweep. A typical rat measured about twelve inches, not counting its tail and, judging from how they felt on my legs, probably weighed four pounds or more.

They made a plentiful food source for rat-eating snakes. I hate rats, but I'm afraid of snakes. If rats infested our bunker, it was certain snakes would come looking for something to eat. I didn't want either one walking or crawling on me.

It wouldn't be prudent to shoot a rat inside our bunker or hooch with an M16. Because none of us had a .45 to use on them—that also would have been a bit too powerful—I asked Bonnie to send me a pellet pistol. She sent a .22-caliber pistol that looked like a Colt revolver. It had a simulated blued-steel frame and plastic wood grain handles. It looked authentic.

It seemed to me at the time that a .22-caliber pellet pistol should do just fine against a rat, even a large rat, especially at a close range of about four to six feet. I was wrong! Those rats were so big and tough that when hit, they would just flinch, then look at me and snarl before taking the cracker or peanut butter I'd left as bait. The snarl lasted only a second and sounded like air escaping from a punctured bicycle tire. One time I could see a rat's long whiskers stretched out a couple of inches beyond its face. It had its lip turned up on the left corner to intentionally expose its teeth. Those rats were obviously too tough to be killed by a pellet pistol, but I managed to kill a couple of them with it anyway.

Terry, who wore a dental plate, took it out at night to sleep. One morning when he got up, he couldn't find his plate. We looked all over the bunker to no avail. Several days later, we found Tom's plate wedged into a corner where it was obvious that a rat had taken it and chewed on it. One afternoon I was talking to a marine when we saw a rat run along a row of sandbags. The marine pulled out his K-bar, threw, and stabbed that rodent, killing and pinning it against a sandbag. It was an impressive display of his knife-throwing talent.

ABOUT TWO-THIRDS OF THE WAY UP the Rockpile, there was a cave. Although it would have been very difficult for anyone to climb to it and take occupancy without being seen, our crew practiced shooting into the cave with several rounds of the Duster's 40-mm guns every few days just to make sure.

Sleeping with your boots on, which is what I did, made it quicker to get up and run to the guns to return fire. That way I didn't have to inspect the inside of my boots before putting my feet inside. The NVA always made their rocket strikes on the base camp at night, so we would wake up and run to the Duster to return fire. It was always just harassing fire because the NVA rarely did much damage. I cannot figure out why they didn't target our OP before striking the base camp, since it had fewer of us to defend it, and would have been easier to overtake.

Monsoon rains are heaviest from June through August, but because Vietnam is located on the equator, it may rain any and every day of the year. Several times we were unable to get down to the river to bathe because of slippery, muddy roads. One time when we hadn't been able to bathe for a couple of weeks, it started to rain; so we all went outside in the rain and soaped up. We were naked, covered in soapsuds, and soaping up our clothes to wash them when the rain stopped. There we were, standing with soap all over us and drying out. I began to feel real crusty and itchy from the drying soap on my body.

It seemed like an hour, but was probably only twenty minutes before it started to rain again, and we were able to wash the soap off our bodies. We lay our shirts and pants out on top of the bunker to let the rain wash out the soap from the fabric. They were pretty stiff when we tried to put them on, so the next time we toughed it out and waited until we could get to the river.

One time I got up during the night to go out to what we called the "shitter," which is the latrine. At night, we have to avoid the use of light because it makes us a target. If we do use a flashlight, we have to put our hand over it to block out all but the tiniest beam of light between the fingers so that we can see where we are going. Well, I was sitting there taking care of business when I felt something crawl across my left leg. It felt lightweight, so light it almost tickled as it came up my inside thigh, over and across the top, and down the outside. I scrambled to locate and turn on my flashlight lying on my right side. I covered it so that only a small crack of light would peak through between my fingers just in time to see a green scorpion two-inches long with its tail straight out behind, going underneath the seat. Its tail and stinger were not over its head, and pointing forward, indicating that it was not feeling threatened and not ready to strike. It may not have felt threatened, but I did. I wasn't about to be stung on my bottom side. That would have been embarrassing to explain at the field hospital. Just like that, I was done. I was up, pants up and out of there in a second and without a light.

My best and worst memories of my life and of Vietnam are from OP Ben.

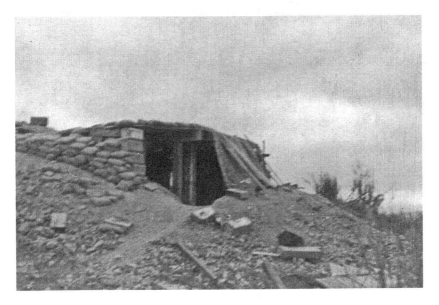

Early stage construction of a bunker

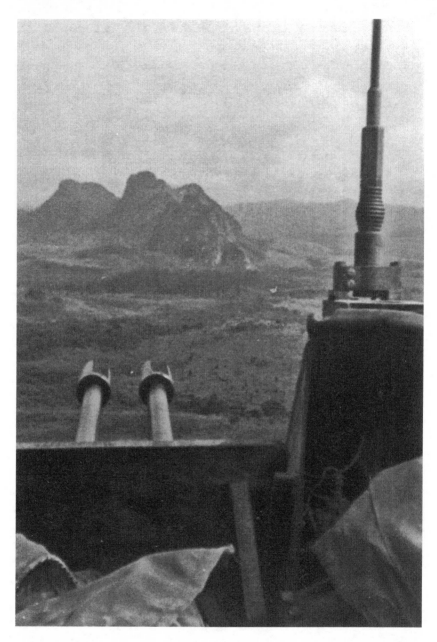

Positioned at OP Ben, the Duster's twin, 40-mm guns point toward the Rockpile.

13

Me and the Guys

During the first few days in Vietnam, I wrote home often, maybe two letters each day to Bonnie and one to my folks. After a of couple weeks, I couldn't think of anything more to write without repeating myself, and it wasn't long before letters were down to two per week to Bonnie and even fewer to Mom and Dad! How many times could I write, "I love you and miss you," before I felt stupid for having nothing to say?

I mean, really? What was I supposed to write? Something like this:

"Hi, I'm doing well; we're learning how to kill Gooks. Well, I've got to go now because we are being hit with another incoming artillery and rocket attack. Bye!"

Most of the letters I did write were to my wife. My mother kept all the letters I wrote to her, and unfortunately, there were not all that many. At the time, I thought I wrote a lot. Reading those letters now, however, I understand why I didn't write much; I had already begun hiding what was going on in my thoughts and in my life.

Instead of writing, I played gin rummy. Leonard, Cefus, Cuba, and I composed the usual players. Combat friends have a special relationship, and these three quickly became my closest friends.

Cuba C. Wright was from Maryland. My friendship with Cuba was deep. He was easy to talk to, and he helped me gain confidence. Cuba was black, and I imagine that is part of what brought us so close together because we spent hours talking about home, family, tradition, and race. We sometimes stayed together during each other's guard duty so that we could talk without others around. I thought our relationship was special, so it would be disappointing to me later, when we would lose contact.

While on guard duty in the small foxhole, sitting close, we exchanged stories. A foxhole is a dug-out piece of earth, or more accurately, a small hole in the ground. The one we occupied near our bunker on OP Ben was about four-feet wide, three-feet deep, and approximately two feet from front to back. We piled up another eight to twelve inches of dirt in front, making it seem another foot deep. That wasn't much room for a single person to spend two or more hours a night in, let alone two men. During the monsoon season, it would fill up with rainwater if we didn't keep it covered with a tarp. Sitting in that foxhole, Cuba told me about his home in Maryland, the sweet potato pie his mamma made, and their family traditions. I told him about my dad playing clarinet and being the leader of a twenty-piece big band during and after World War II. We whispered and watched the darkness. We talked about religion, and discrimination, and the atrocities committed by our nation against its own people. We marveled at the stars and all of God's creation, even though I don't believe we included Vietnam in our appreciation.

LEONARD BRUSKI, WHOM WE ALSO called Rufus, really liked the spaghetti and meatballs in a case of C-rations. Every time we opened a new case, he would call dibs on the spaghetti and meatballs. Each meal had a can of the main course, spaghetti and meatballs, ham and lima beans (also known as ham and mother fuckers), scrambled eggs, and others. Also in the box was a small can called a B-2 Unit, offering crackers and jelly, muffin or pound cake, a small amount of toilet paper, and a pack of four cigarettes. We used that small can, the B-2 Unit, as a stove to heat the meal. We cut off the top and then cut half way around the edge at the top and bottom so that the side could be pushed in toward the back to allow the larger can to sit on top. To heat the meal we used either large artillery gunpowder or C-4 plastic explosive that we lit with a match. Both burned extremely hot, but the C-4 was much hotter. When it burned, it put out a ball of white light that glittered and sparkled until it had all burned away.

By now that can of spaghetti was probably forty-five years old, produced for World War II. It was filled to the brim, a congealed clump of cold spaghetti. Leonard broke off a piece of C-4 and put it in the small bottom can, set his can of spaghetti and meatballs on top, and lit the C-4. We saw bright light and sparks, and we could hear the roar of the C-4 burning. The can of spaghetti started to shake and wobble. A sort of soft sound built up, like the sound of a mortar leaving its tube, only far away, maybe like a distant muzzle. Then Leonard's spaghetti shot up into the air like a red, jelly-filled rocket. Leonard grabbed his helmet, yelling, "My spaghetti!" He chased it, trying to catch it as it fell. The memory of that flying spaghetti will stay with me forever.

Dennis Ramsey, Cefus, came from a rural area in Tennessee on the Tobacco Road, very close to where the movie by the same name was filmed, according to Dennis. He had an authentic southern drawl, with slow, stretched-out words that all just sort of ran together. He could turn a whole sentence into one word.

I don't know if *Cefus* was a name Dennis used at home or just since arriving in the army, but it seemed to fit. I guess it was his Tennessee blood that made it necessary for him to make the rest of us shut up and let him listen to The Grand Ol' Opry. Every Saturday evening the single radio we had was tuned to

AFBN, the Armed Forces Broadcasting Network.

I can still hear him now, with his slow southern drawl: "Now euen boys, be quiat fo a bit, so I-cn lisn ta theus." Translation: "You guys shut up so I can hear this."

Then, the rest of the night, we would all mockingly talk with his southern accent.

Dennis entertained us with stories about living in Tennessee on Tobacco Road. He kept us spellbound describing how he ran moonshine to local areas for delivery.

Len, on the other hand, smoked and chewed on a cigar that was sent to him in the mail from home while he described twenty-foot high snowdrifts and the shoveled tunnels he dug at his home in Alpena, Michigan.

There were others: Andy Soo, "Shorty" Thomas, Terry Holmes, and "Zique" McHenry. Holmes filled the spot created when Soo rotated back to the world. Holmes was short, about five-foot-four and small framed, but he talked about picking up on girls using his favorite pick up line, "I'm not very big, but I've got a cute way of rollin' on and off."

When Cuba left to return home, his replacement, Sgt. McHenry, joined us. McHenry often talked about living in the Bronx of New York. One time while at OP Ben, a chaplain came up to visit those of us on the hill. We were standing in front of our bunker and could see Highway 9 below. While we talked to the chaplain, we saw an unusually long convoy traveling on the road. Zique, talking in his usual New York accent and using his most common adjective, said, "Look at the size of that fucking convoy!"

Then realizing the expletive he had just used, he said, "Oh, excuse me Father!"

The chaplain just laughed and said, "Well, I guess it's a pretty sexy convoy, huh?"

Swearing was used with much emphasis and regularity in the army. In Vietnam, it was in almost every sentence. There was a two-word phrase that was used to explain our attitude and end almost every story, no matter what the subject of conversation. When talking about the U.S. Army, the Marine Corps, and especially Vietnam, and women (except when talking about your own or someone else's mother), the final statement was always an emphatic, "Fuck it!"

"Fuck'n-A" indicated a positive response.

My parents did not use swear words. I had heard the *F*-word and possibly even used it a time or two, but never around my parents. My first day at the induction center, I heard it used several times, along with several other exclamations. It was a bit shocking to hear all that profanity—and often in just one sentence! At first, I was uncomfortable with hearing it used continuously, but it wasn't long before I was using it regularly myself. I guess the chaplain had heard it all, too.

In Vietnam, it didn't take long to learn that if you became attached to someone, it wouldn't be long before they would be gone. Friends finished their tour of duty or they got injured or killed. Either way, they were gone, and you were left there alone. It was better not to get to know anyone—or at least not care about anyone because they would just leave you. When I think of the people I lost while there, I know I was lucky. There were just the five of us as the crew on our Duster, and we never lost anyone to a combat casualty although there were guys who finished their tour of duty and went home. It wasn't just combat buddies who left, either. It was girlfriends and wives. Somebody in the battery was always getting a "Dear John" letter.

The ones I mourn are the ones I didn't know by name—the marines who were killed as they ran into harm's way, the ones we put on medevac choppers. I mourn the kid at Camp J.J. Carroll who was shot by a sniper while at the river filling a water tank. I mourn Lan, the Vietnamese boy I befriended. It should have been me who died in Vietnam; it would have been so much easier than carrying this yoke of shame and survivor guilt.

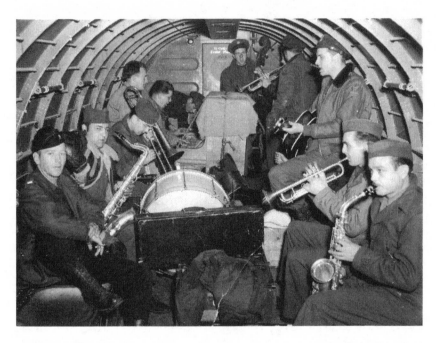

Blaylock's father, front right, with his band on a plane flight headed for a gig

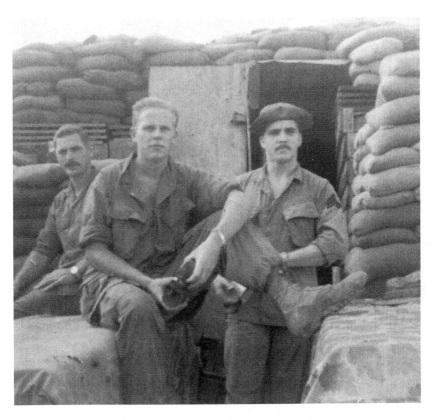

Leonard, from left, Bill Blaylock, and George

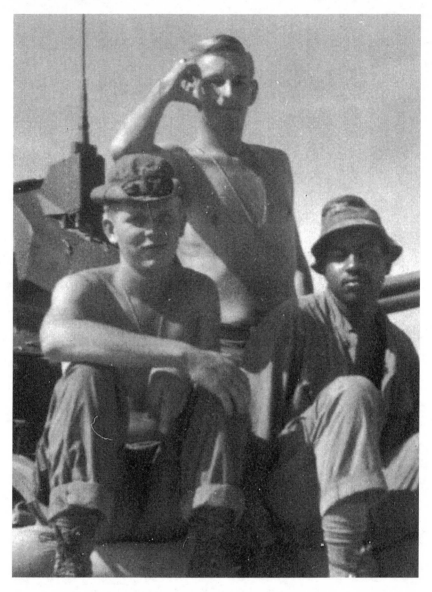

Dennis, from left, Bill Blaylock, and Cuba on the Duster

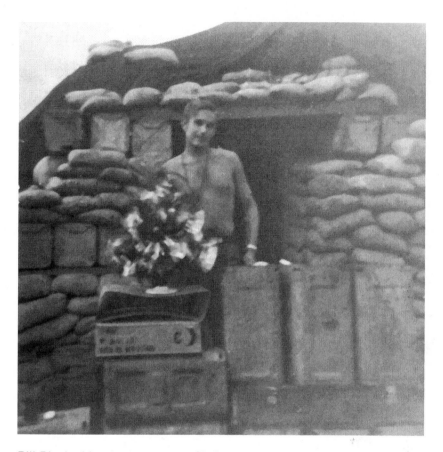

Bill Blaylock's parents sent a Christmas tree to Vietnam as part of a December care package.

14

War at OP Ben

I realized the war was real while stationed at OP Ben. It was late April, and I had been in the country a month and a half. I was on guard duty, crouched in the small dugout. Guard duty was usually a two- to three-hour shift spent staying still and not making any noise. The purpose was to listen and look for anything unusual or anything moving that should not be moving. Usually, the most difficult part of being on guard duty was not falling asleep. The next most difficult part of guard duty was lighting a cigarette without allowing any light from the lighter to give away my position. Otherwise, I could become a target. Also difficult was cupping my hands over the tip of the cigarette to hide the glow. When my shift was over, I crawled over and woke up my relief person.

One night, I saw two faint and small red and green lights about twenty yards away, just about where the perimeter wire would be if I had been able to see it. They disappeared, and then I saw them again. They disappeared and then reappeared again. I wasn't sure I believed what I was seeing. It was so dark; there was no moon, and the sky had a thick heavy cloud cover. Whispering into the microphone and turning down the speaker volume, I called my sergeant on the two-way radio. He notified the marines a few yards away, and one of them brought over a sniper rifle that had a "Starlight" scope attached. The marine didn't see anyone, but he thought something didn't look right. We put up luminary flares from one of the marine mortars to get a better look, but there was no movement. The next morning we found the perimeter wire had been cut several times right where I had seen the lights. I knew then—and I was resolved to the fact—that I was going to die in this place so far from home. From that time forward, I always slept on my back; I felt less vulnerable. On my back, I could respond quicker to any threat. I did not know it then, but it would be years before I could sleep in any other position.

OUR BATTERY WAS PRIMARILY RESPONSIBLE for morning mine sweeps to clear Highway 9 for daily traffic use. It was May 6, 1968; a sniper on the road to Khe Sanh fired a round so close to my left ear that I could hear the wind as it zinged past. I knew that one was for me. I, myself, had personally been shot at for the first time. I had been in firefights before. The first and second ones were on my second day in the country as part of the convoy to Camp Carroll. Nevertheless, this was the first bullet that I knew was intended for me. I heard it and knew it was close.

We were on our daily mine sweep, traveling west on Highway 9 from the Rockpile, toward Khe Sanh about nine miles away. We expected to meet halfway with a team from Khe Sanh. We had been on the road for a little over an hour. The sun was bright and the day already warm. The tall green grass and dark green trees of the jungle contrasted the terracotta red clay soil.

Everything was peaceful as we slowly rode along at the pace set by the marines walking ahead. They carried metal detectors with headphone listening devices attached. They swept the width of the road, listening for the sound made by the detector when it gets close to a metal object. They needed the headphones to hear the metal detectors' audible signal over the noise of our heavy mechanized equipment not far behind. The only sound I could hear in my gunner's seat was the noise of our Duster's motor and the sound of its steel tracks clanking against the rugged steel teeth of the drive gears. For me, the biggest concern with the mine sweeps was when we stopped. Stopping made us a stationary target. Even though we moved slowly, at least we were moving. Even if the VC planted a false device for us to find, it meant we would have to stop, dig it up, and then determine if it needed to be detonated or discarded. The longer we stopped, the better target we were.

Suddenly, gunfire erupted. The entire force sprang into action. The marines with the metal detectors hit the dirt and crawled to the edge of the road for cover. The rifle squad walking behind dropped to the ground and returned fire into the trees about forty or fifty yards away on the right side of the road. Marines in the truck behind us jumped out and took cover positions from behind the truck to fire back. Others ran to positions at the edge of the road in a ditch and behind brush to conceal their position. Cuba and I immediately turned our guns in the direction of where the marines were shooting and began to fire the twin 40-mm rounds. I saw trees exploding and branches flying to the ground as our rounds exploded against them.

Zzzing! I heard the sound of a bullet pass by my left ear. Time didn't stand still. It sped up, and my rage increased exponentially. Yelling into the microphone of my helmet, I shouted, "Those bastards are trying to kill me."

Cuba didn't respond; we just kept firing and doing our job. Then the shooting stopped. Just as suddenly as it had started, it stopped. That's the way it always was. There wasn't any tapering off; it was always instantly on or off. I lived in a constant state of preparedness and on hyper-alert. We waited while a small patrol went out to check the area for evidence of enemy kills. I never learned what the results were from the patrol, but it didn't matter to me. When the patrol returned, we loaded up and continued the mine sweep of the road. Other than commenting on how sudden the whole thing started and stopped, we rarely talked about it.

It wasn't long before feeling close rounds became a fairly regular event, and I did not write about it in my photo album anymore. I was the gunner on the Duster and possibly the first target, although the two cannoneers standing in the turret and leaning over the side to retrieve more ammo made excellent targets, too.

Our camp regularly took incoming artillery fire, and we returned it. We were often attacked by snipers and were involved in some small ambushes on our daily road sweeps for mines. Fortunately and amazingly, none of us were ever seriously injured in any of these attacks. Once, we were recognized for our swift and accurate return of fire during an incoming rocket attack that resulted in significant damage to the enemy.

OTHER SIMILAR EVENTS TRANSPIRED, but I did not write about them then. Today I wish I had. Perhaps my reason for not writing was embarrassment. I was embarrassed that I might be trying to glorify myself or my actions, so I just didn't write anymore, as I had when I first started keeping our album. However, some combat encounters stayed with me, etched in my mind forever, even though I did not record them in Vietnam.

THE INCIDENT THAT HAUNTS ME to this day occurred in early June or early July 1968. We were to assist a company of marines pinned down in a ravine in an ambush somewhere on Highway 9, east of our location at the Rockpile. They were taking fire from both sides of the road. The river was located on my left side, and the area was full of heavy vegetation. Up the ravine and across the river onto the other side, the ground was dense with dark green trees and brush. The shallow ditch alongside the ravine on my right did not provide much protection from the enemies' elevated firing position. The marines took heavy casualties. They needed extra firepower, so they could retrieve their dead and wounded.

Air support was called, bringing two F4 Phantoms dropping napalm and high explosive ordinance on enemy positions on the riverside of the road. The bombs were so close that their shock wave rattled our enormously heavy Duster. Breathing was difficult because napalm briefly sucked the oxygen out of the air. I felt the heat on the left side of my face, and then I felt the wind rush against my right side as the oxygenated air was being drawn to the fire to fuel the napalm.

Our job entailed driving into the kill zone to put out as much firepower as possible, so the marines could clear out the area. We were the lead Duster and took the right side of the road, firing up into the ravine. The other Duster took the left, firing on the area between the road and the river that had been napalmed by the air force F4 Phantoms. The injured would be loaded onto our Dusters for a ride to the landing zone (LZ) where they could be evacuated by helicopter.

Soo drove us into the kill zone with bodies of marines, dead and injured still littering the road ahead. Marines crouched low and close to the Duster protecting their blind side. Len fired the M60 mounted on the back of the turret, and the marines assaulted with their M16 and M79 grenade launchers as we drove in.

I can still see the bodies of marines on the road. My worst fear was that we would run over our own men, whether dead or wounded. I prayed that the marines moving along our side would be able to pull the bodies clear of the tracks. We moved forward, positioning to fire.

The enemy continued to fire down on us as we moved in. Only seconds after firing our 40-mm guns at their full rate capacity of 240 rounds per minute, the enemy fire stopped. We continued to fire at everything, so they wouldn't have a chance to rise up and continue their attack. We sprayed rounds all over the ravine not knowing exactly where the enemy positions actually were. I could smell and see smoke from small grass fires in the ravine. I smelled the burnt gunpowder.

An injured marine was lifted up on the side of the Duster. Leonard and I held him there while we drove him and others back down the road to an LZ to be flown to a field hospital. He lay in a poncho sling covered in blood and that damn red-earth mud. He suffered entry wounds all over his body, his legs, arms, face, and torso except where a flak vest provided a modicum of protection. The vest had its own tears, showing the interior fabric. It was hard to tell where the mud stopped and the blood began. I presumed he had been hit by a grenade or land mine to have so many entry wounds. The medic pressed bandages under his clothing trying to stop the bleeding. Two morphine syringes were pinned to his left shirt collar. Combat medics used single-dose morphine in squeeze tubes with a needle attached. Each time one was dispensed to an injured warrior, it was stuck in his shirt collar. The needle bent over, so it would stay in place, signaling to medevac and hospital attendants how much morphine he had been given in the field.

In the midst of all the commotion, shooting continued back in the ravine as marines advanced to pursue and engage the enemy. The noise level was so intense it was difficult to concentrate. Gunfire rang out over the sound of shouts, the noise of the motor, and the loud squeaking of the Duster grinding metal-on-metal along our tracks.

Smoke rose from the burning jungle where the napalm hit. The drops deployed a devastating inferno of fury. The distinct smell of cordite from the burnt gunpowder drew thick in the air. I remember every sensation vividly, as if it were happening right now. Then for me everything went silent, as though I had suddenly gone deaf.

The scene became worse when the young marine loaded onto our Duster held up his right arm. He displayed a right hand just barely attached. Only a thin layer of skin connected his hand to his arm. I saw bone and flesh in plain sight. A tourniquet stemmed the flow of blood. In spite of it all, the injured marine was able to make us laugh—a flicker of humanity amid grotesque violence. "I guess I'll have to learn how to jack off with my left hand!" he said.

Just as suddenly as the sounds stopped for me, the noise of the war all instantly returned, and we began moving backward along the dirt road to a freshly cut LZ to deliver our evacuees.

Sometimes, I laugh when I think of this story, and sometimes I get choked up and cry. The trauma to that marine and trauma to all of us that day was sad, funny, and disturbing all at the same time. I presumed it was the morphine in him, but it may have been his own brave humor that allowed him to make such a funny statement, working through his own pain and misfortune to get him—and us—through the ordeal. I pray that he made it. I wish I knew his name!

Every time I see or hear an ambulance, I see that marine and re-live that day. Every time I pass an accident, I remember that marine and re-live that day. I remember all those marines, all those bodies, that whole day. Every time I hear a helicopter, I see that marine going to his medevac. In my mind, I see all the mud and blood. I smell the burnt gunpowder. I see and smell the smoke. I hear the yelling of scared and excited soldiers alongside marines tangling with the orders of officers, each and all trying to communicate to anyone who could hear or would listen. I hear the screams of pain and calls for help.

This day repeats over and over, year after year. Rarely a day goes by when I won't confront a circumstantial trigger, surfacing the mental pictures of that marine and that day of infamy. When I remember or talk about this firefight, only occasionally do I maintain composure. Most often, I do not.

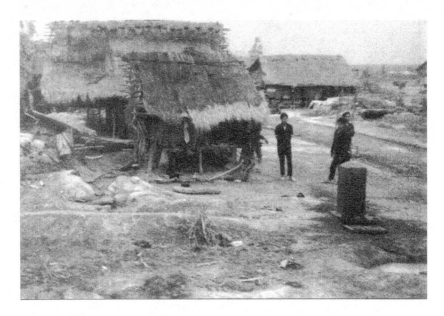

Vietnam village of Cam Lo

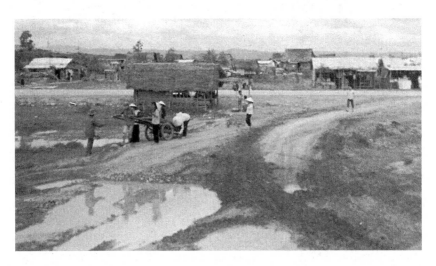

The village of Cam Lo and surrounding area

15

War Isn't Always Hell

In June 1968, I developed a severe cough and felt weak, so the sergeant sent me to sick call at the Camp Rockpile Medical Clinic. Late in the afternoon a doctor finally diagnosed me with pneumonia. An hour later, I joined a convoy to Dong Ha, and then a chopper with about four other guys flying to Da Nang.

With the slow convoy and getting a late start, it was about 2130 hours before we boarded the chopper to Da Nang. The clock passed 2200 when we arrived at the Da Nang hospital. Rain poured most of the day, but when we got off the chopper, it seemed to be coming down extra hard and heavy. The chopper set down a few paces from the entrance to the emergency check-in. The ground was slushy with thick mud, making it difficult to get to the entrance.

The emergency check-in was a large canvas tent that connected to a conventional structure. The entrance side had a large flap that pulled down to help keep out the wind, dust, and rain. Secure tie-downs ensured the structure could withstand the turbulence of helicopter rotor blades.

None of us required a stretcher, and we were able to walk in ourselves, but it was difficult to get any attention. A row of folding chairs lined one side of the canvas tent, and someone told us to have a seat. I was in the second chair from the left. The five of us had been sitting there for only a few minutes, wrapped in wet ponchos, when an army WAC major walked up. One of the guys attempted to stand up to salute her. She gently reached out, touched his shoulder, and said, "No. Don't get up or salute!"

After a short pause, in the gentlest and most motherly voice I have ever heard, she said, "Have you boys had dinner or something to eat?"

Almost in unison, we responded, "No Ma'am!"

Instantly, she rose up, pivoted in place, and barked out, "Get these men some dinner—right now!"

I don't think that the words had cleared her mouth when about a dozen hospital personnel ran off to the mess hall. Within a couple of minutes, each of us had a tray full of food. Hot food! Good food! The hospital was going to be like R&R. Portions spread far enough for at least four more people to eat. Best of all, nothing in front of us was a C-ration.

The major turned back to face us and in her gentle and caring voice again, she said, "Now you boys try to relax, and we will be with you in just a few minutes."

She turned and walked away. That was the last I saw of her, but she was right; it wasn't long before we were all seen by doctors and taken to a comfortable bed.

The beds actually had mattresses and white linen, even a pillow. The pillow was an inflatable bag that I deflated and stuffed inside my shirt and took with me when discharged from the hospital. It was a lot more comfortable than using a rolled-up towel or my steel helmet.

Each time I think of this story, I laugh at the instantaneous changes in demeanor the WAC major went through and how everyone jumped when she shouted out her orders. That was sure funny to watch.

WHEN I WAS A KID, MY FATHER CUT my hair with an old pair of shiny chrome clippers that constantly needed lubricating with three-in-one oil. When the handles were squeezed together, the cutting edges moved across each other to cut the hair.

Since the same kind of hand-operated clipper was available to us at OP Ben, the crew decided that I should be the designated barber. There was some joking around about my doing the haircuts because I had told them that, before the army, I had worked at a mortuary. I was not a mortician; that was true. I didn't tell them, but I did not do any barber work either. Nevertheless, I told them I had cut the hair for our customers, and that's where I got my experience. I joked that I was pretty skilled at it because I never got a complaint. The complaints I got while cutting the crews' hair only came when I told them, "Lay perfectly still on your back!"

A walkway we built led to the entrance of our bunker. It was about eight- to ten-feet long and stacked with sandbags to three-feet high on each side. This constituted my barber shop. My customers or victims would sit on a 40-mm ammo can, nicely positioned for me to cut their hair.

I began cutting Leonard's hair. As usual, it was getting to be a warm day. Dennis and Cuba were standing several feet away in front of us, watching. Suddenly, one of them started yelling at us, "Watch out, down by your leg!" Both Leonard and I looked down and saw a huge centipede crawling out from between some sandbags and stretching out toward my leg. We couldn't see its full length yet, but its body was about three-quarters of an inch wide, with legs extending beyond that. It had front feelers more than an inch long. It was black with a bright orange stripe running all the way down the top of its back. We both jumped out of the way.

I ran inside the bunker to get some bug repellent. When I came out, Leonard was trying to poke at the creature with his knife, the weapon he bought from a marine and kept strapped to his leg. I squeezed the can to squirt bug repellent on the centipede. The bug juice didn't seem to hurt it any, but the centipede didn't like it. In fact, it seemed only to make it mad. The centipede finally crawled out from the sandbags and started to run away from the bunker in the direction of where Dennis and Cuba had been standing. Leonard continued slashing at it on the ground with his knife, until he had finally dismembered it so many times that it stopped moving. When we got all the pieces back together, it was about a foot long.

ON THE FOURTH OF JULY, our battery put on quite a party. The mess hall at Camp Rockpile sent up to our position some canisters containing real steaks, baked potatoes, and macaroni salad. The food was put into insulated containers similar to a metal ice chest, loaded onto a helicopter, and then flown to our hilltop. The chopper slowed and briefly hovered about twenty feet above our position while a crewman dropped out the canisters. They hit the ground and fortunately didn't break open. We inspected the slightly dented gifts that had just been dropped off only to find the steaks and potatoes now thoroughly mixed together, and extra well-mixed macaroni salad in the other. Along with the new food, we had five cases of soda pop on hand and three cases of beer. We were stationed on an observation post, so items that we normally would have had to purchase from a commissary were given to us, including the free soda and beer.

The steaks and potatoes were hot. So were the soda and beer. We didn't care; it all tasted pretty good to us. Although I had enjoyed beer when stationed at Fort Sill, and a few times since, I decided to hold off. One of the marines, Cuba, and I stuck to drinking cola. The rest of the marine squad, about ten guys, and the remaining three of our crew, all drank beer. I don't know if they liked the beer or drank it because it was there and free.

We started our celebration at 1130 and ended it at about 1930. We had a terrific time. I was glad that I had only had soda because it was a lot more fun watching the drunks stumble around. How fortunate we weren't attacked that night.

Our observation post was about a mile away from the camp, and it was considered to be a dangerous drive between the two locations. We were pretty much left alone to do what we wanted as long as we showed up in the morning for our road mine sweep. My experience in Vietnam left me with an impression that there was a lack of supervision from officers, not just in our unit, but also in the oversight of the Vietnam War itself. Officers had, for the most part, lost control of many actions of enlisted men. There weren't any officers who wanted to take the drive in a jeep up the hill to visit our position. That's probably why the helicopter didn't land, but instead, dropped the food containers to us.

ONE TIME WHEN LEN WAS DRIVER, probably early August, we had a staff sergeant riding in the observer's seat. We had just completed a morning mine sweep. For the return trip from the end of the mine sweep, we could drive back as fast as we wanted. The Duster's transmission had a two-speed gearbox, low and high. Len liked to floor the throttle in low gear and then speed shift into the high gear, which made the duster leap forward like a race car shifting into its next gear. The staff sergeant was sitting high in the seat with his body well above the open hatch. Len performed his usual high-speed shifting technique; however, this time he missed the high gear and, instead, went into reverse. The Duster immediately slammed to a stop and started to back up. Len slammed on the brakes, but it was too late. That staff sergeant flew out of the Duster and onto the dirt road in front. The cord on his helmet stretched out straight. The cord pulled out from its helmet connection and came whipping back up to the Duster, slamming against and ricocheting off the front of the turret. It was funny at the time, but Len didn't think so when he got a severe ass chewing from the sergeant.

"You're not back at home driving a race car," he said. "Knock that shit off."

IN VIETNAM, WE DIDN'T HAVE FLUSH TOILETS, and the outhouses we built ourselves. At Camp J.J. Carroll, our Headquarters Battery had recently built a new ten-hole latrine. It was constructed so that one half of a fifty-five-gallon barrel cut around its diameter could be placed underneath each toilet seat. Everyday someone, usually a new guy, would be assigned to burn the shitter. The procedure for this assignment was to open the lids behind each hole and slide out the container. Then several feet away from the outhouse, the assigned soldier would pour enough diesel fuel into the container to cover the waste and light the diesel on fire.

One day the first sergeant, who was proud and happy about his new latrine, called over some kid new in the country, and told him to go burn the shitter. About twenty minutes later, the first sergeant came out of his office and saw his new shitter fully engulfed in flames. He yelled and chased that poor kid all over the compound, threatening the FNG (fucking new guy) with court martial and screaming things about his mother and family with every obscenity he could think of. The first sergeant would have surely hurt him badly if he had caught him. As I remember it, everyone else just watched and laughed as the chase ensued around the burning latrine.

WHEN RETURNING TO OP BEN one morning from the daily road-clearing mine sweep, we rode the Duster with six marines who were also camped on the observation post at that time. The road back up the hill to our OP was a twisty, uneven strip of dirt from where the tracks and tires of our vehicles had crushed down the natural grass and vegetation. To the side of the road, grass and weeds sprouted dry about three-feet tall. Riding up the road and coming around a slight bend, someone spotted a wild boar sow and several piglets in the tall grass about thirty yards off the road to our left.

The black sow and piglets stood in harsh contrast against the tall yellowish, wheat-colored dry grass they were grazing in. The sow was a little less than three-feet tall and approximately four and a half feet long. The three piglets were no more than ten to twelve inches long. Lazily snorting and rooting through the tall grass, they posed no threat to us. They didn't seem to be bothered by our movement or the loud clanking sounds of our heavy machinery.

If only they had run!

"Hey look over there, a wild pig," someone said. "Let's shoot it."

Almost instantly, we all opened up with our M16 rifles. Dennis, George, Leonard, Shorty, the six marines, and I, were all firing. Hot brass bullet casings flew everywhere including against my neck and down the back of my flack jacket and then down past my collar. I was so jacked up that I didn't feel the hot brass as it hit against my neck and fell down my back until I stopped to reload. It felt so good to shoot that stupid damn pig. Rage took control of my body and mind. I spent a full magazine of ammo with the selector switch on full auto with only two squeezes of the trigger.

I looked down to eject the empty magazine cartridge. I inserted a full one to fire again, but when I looked up to find the target, nothing was there—no sow, no piglets, no nothing. Just patches of flattened down, blood-saturated and spattered, dry grass.

We didn't stop to inspect our kill; we just continued on up the road, shouting, whooping, and hollering out, "Yoo-hoo, yeah, right on"—a victory over that "stupid, fucking Vietnamese pig, its useless environment, and this whole God-damned country."

We briefly felt satisfaction. None of us spoke of it again.

THEN THERE WAS THE TIME that I shot Leonard. We were at Camp J.J. Carroll. It was close to dusk. I was walking with Shorty and playing with the pellet pistol that my wife had sent to shoot rats inside the bunker. I was doing the usual cowboy show-off stuff, trying to spin it with my finger in the trigger guard. For some stupid reason, I pointed it in Len's direction and said some dumb thing like "hands up." Suddenly it just went off and the .22-caliber pellet hit Len in the arm.

He yelled and got out of his chair faster than lightning, starting toward me. I couldn't just stand there and let him punch me with those great big hands of his. I mean he had enormous, tough hands, with fingers as large as sausages. I began to run, and we went quite a way, nearly to the south end of the camp, before we both were too tired to continue. He accepted my apology; we both laughed and walked back to the hooch.

TO RELAX OUR BODY AND MIND, we drank beer that we got from the base camp, or Gook booze we would purchase from the locals along the road after a morning mine sweep. They tried to sell anything and everything they thought we wanted. We always had to inspect the bottles for ground glass in the bottoms, before drinking. Getting a "buzz on" two or three times a week, playing cards, and writing letters home was the best pastime. Guys from other Duster crews and marines said that getting "high" was better because it did not leave them with a hangover the next morning. I tried to see if their theory was true one evening by going to another crew's hooch to smoke marijuana. After a couple of draws off the joint, I decided it wasn't for me. I went back to my own hooch to have a drink with Cefus and Rufus.

IN EARLY JANUARY, 1969, WE PROVIDED security for a Seabee unit extracting rock from the Cam Lo River and crushing it to make gravel for the roads in our area. We spotted a large lizard on the north side of the river sunning itself on a rock. We watched it lying flat, and still on the rock about one hundred twenty yards from our position. It was about three and a half feet long from head to tail, a sort of pale green and gray in color, with short legs.

The north side of the river was considered Charlie's territory, a dangerous place to be, but that was where the lizard was resting. We passed the word that we were going to fire a couple of rounds with an M16, so everyone would know it was friendly fire.

Crack. Jeff fired, hit, and killed the lizard with one shot.

While he went down to the river and swam across to retrieve his hunt, we intently watched at the ready to protect him. Later, back at our bunker, he skinned the carcass and laid it out to dry on the cardboard from an empty case of C-rations. Later he stretched and mounted the skin over his helmet with the tail hanging down about two feet behind. It was impressive and made an impressive camouflage. He wore it with pride for the rest of his tour.

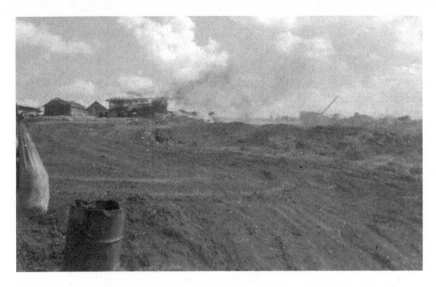

The first sergeant's new latrine becomes engulfed in fire.

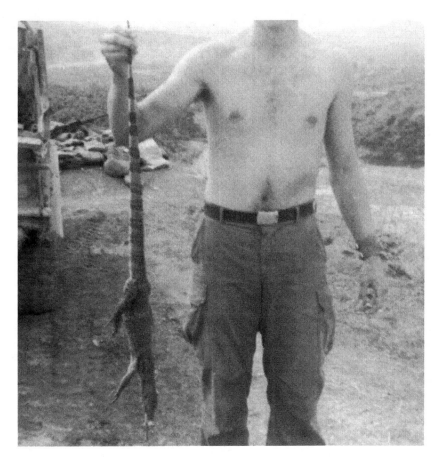

Encroaching into "Charlie territory," Jeff shot this lizard, and then he mounted the skin over his helmet with the tail hanging down about two feet behind.

16

Winding Down

I hadn't been in the country long before I began to notice that the predominant topic anyone talked about was "getting back to the world." Going home was the primary motivation for survival. Every time I met someone, if they didn't tell me first, it was courtesy for me to ask.

"How long you got in the 'Nam?"

Their response would be measured in "days left to go in country." I earned considerable commiseration and laughter when I replied, "360 and a wake up!"

Occasionally I would encounter someone who would respond with, "I'm a short timer: twenty-nine and a wake up!"

A short-timer was anyone who had thirty days or fewer remaining in the country. Even attaining double-digit status— ninety-nine or fewer—was monumental. Short-timers employed phrases to emphasize the brevity of their tour. I found my favorite line when I heard, "I'm so short I have to look up to see down."

We made short-timer sticks, also known as swagger sticks that we carried around proclaiming our limited time left in "the Nam." The sticks consisted of pieces of wooden dowel no more than two-feet long, ends featuring either the front or the back of a bullet cartridge cut in half. The stick resembled a long bullet.

Cuba returned to "The World" in September of 1968 and found himself stationed at Fort Bliss, Texas for the remainder of his enlistment.

On December 18, 1968, we abandoned Camp J.J. Carroll. We destroyed and burned the buildings. Our battery received orders to provide security for a Seabees unit located a short distance down Highway 9, east of the old Camp Carroll and toward Dong Ha, close to the Song Cam Lo River that ran parallel to Highway 9 in most of that area of Cam Lo Province.

The Seabees had bulldozers and other heavy equipment. They could dig out and fortify perimeter guard locations around the entire camp. They dug out holes three-feet deep and six-feet wide for guard bunkers, easily allowing three men to move comfortably and watch their assigned field of security. The bunkers had large timbers behind them and an overhang to provide protection from enemy fire as well as from weather. They pushed up a mound of dirt about eight feet high around the entire camp to make it extra difficult for enemy soldiers to assault. They built three guard towers at least twenty-feet high, large enough to accommodate a machine gun and three men.

However, it didn't end there. The Seabees also built us above-ground hooches, with sandbags filled and placed protectively around the structure. They even built us a shower with heated water. The Seabees' primary function, as I understood it, was to build and improve roads in the area. All we had to do was provide perimeter guard duty, and during the day we would escort them and their equipment to the river and provide security there while they dug up river rock, took it back to camp, and crushed it to make gravel to put down on the roads.

The first time we saw eight-year-old Lan was at the river where the Seabees got their rock. As he approached, he did not seem to be any threat, wearing only his dirty torn shirt and short pants.

Each day Lan came to our location. He would spend the day hanging out and talking with us. This kid had experienced more trauma than anyone should at his young age. Lan would hang out with us all day long, drinking our warm Coca Cola, when we had it, and smoking our American cigarettes. He liked Marlboro the best, then either Kool or Salem menthols. Lan would let us know if there were any enemy movements in the area. He told us that if he wasn't present some day, we should be extra careful. Then he'd say, "VC number ten fuckin' thousand!"

He was a good kid. We all wanted to take him home to America and adopt him. When I told him that, he said, "No, GI, you go your home. I stay mine."

We always made sure he was fed and had some C-rations to eat. I don't know where or how he is now, but I hope and pray that he was able to survive the war and maybe even remember some of the time he spent with those GIs. When I would eventually leave the Nam, I would remember him by the photographs I took.

IN A LETTER DATED DECEMBER 2, 1968, to my parents, I had copied a poem that had been in *Stars and Stripes*:

VIETNAM

Across the Pacific Ocean,
Vietnam was the spot.
Ten thousand miles from you,
The spot that God forgot.
We work, we sweat,
It's more than we can stand.
We're not supposed to be convicts,
But defenders of our land.
We're members of U.S. Armed Forces
Getting very little pay.

Defending people with millions
For a lousy two and a half a day.
Living with our memories
Waiting to be with our gals.
Hoping all the while
They haven't married our pals.
Nobody knows we're living,
No one gives a damn.
At home we were forgotten,
We belong to Uncle Sam.
When we die and go to Heaven
We'll hear St. Peter yell.
Let the boys from Vietnam through,
For they have spent their time in Hell.

When I sent this letter to my parents, I wasn't quite a short-timer, but I had less than one hundred days left of my tour of duty, ninety-three days to be exact.

I don't think I was trying to make a statement. I just thought the poem sounded cool and made us look tough, like warriors. All my letters home were positive. I didn't talk about negative things, and I didn't complain about conditions or attitudes. I talked about the weather and all the rain during the monsoon season, but without complaint. I was already suppressing and storing away emotion and trauma. I never wrote home about firefights, and I didn't talk about them after I got home.

A form letter circulated among the troops. It was funny to me at the time, but in retrospect, it was amazingly intuitive. I sent it home in a letter to my wife and parents about three weeks before my scheduled departure from Vietnam, the middle of February. I didn't know anything about PTSD back then, but upon reflection, I can now see that this author was alluding to problems for returning veterans.

Dear Civilian, Friend, Draft Dodgers, Etc.

In the very near future the undersigned will once more be in your midst, dehydrated, and demoralized to take his place again as a human being with the well-known forms of freedom and justice for all; engaging in Life, Liberty and the somewhat delayed Pursuit of Happiness. In making your joyous preparations to welcome him back into organized society, you might take certain steps to make allowances for the crude environment, which has been his miserable lot for the past twelve months. In other words, he might be a little Asiatic from Vietnameseitis and Overseasitis and should and handled with care. Do not be alarmed if he was infected with all forms of rare tropical diseases. A little time in the "Land of the Big PX" will cure this malady.

Therefore, show no alarm if he insists on carrying a weapon to the dinner table, looks around for his steel pot when offered a chair, or wakes you up in the middle of the night for guard duty. Keep cool when he pours gravy on his dessert at dinner or mixes peaches with his Seagram's VO. Pretend not to notice if he eats with his fingers instead of silverware and prefers C-rations to steak. Abstain from saying anything about powdered eggs, dehydrated potatoes, fried rice, fresh milk, or ice cream. Do not be alarmed if he should jump from the dinner table to rush to the garbage can to wash his dish with a toilet brush. After all, this has been his standard.

When in his daily conversation he utters such things as "Xin Loi" and "Choi Oi," just be patient, and simply leave quickly and calmly if by some chance he utters "Di Di" with an irritated look on his face because it means no less than "Get the hell out of here." Do not let it shake you up if he picks up the phone and yells "iron hand, sir" or says, "out here" for goodbye, or simply shouts, "working."

Never ask why the Jones' son held a higher rank than he did and by no means mention the term "xtend." Pretend not to notice if, at a restaurant, he calls the waitress, "number one girl" and uses his hat for an ashtray. He will probably keep listening for the sounds of "in-coming." If he does, comfort him, for he is still reminiscing. Be especially watchful when he is in the presence of a woman – especially a beautiful woman.

Above all, keep in mind that beneath that tanned and rugged exterior there is a heart of gold (the only thing of value he has left). Treat him with kindness, tolerance and an occasional fifth of good liquor, and you will be able to rehabilitate that which was once (and now is a hallow shell of) the happy-go-lucky guy you once knew and loved.

Last, but by no means least, send no more mail to the APO, fill the refrigerator with beer, get the civvies out of the mothballs, fill the car with gas, and get the women and children off the streets—BECAUSE THE KID IS COMING HOME!

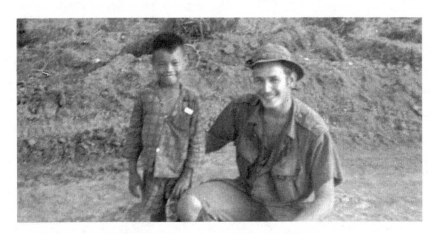

Eight-year-old Vietnamese boy, Lan, with Bill Blaylock

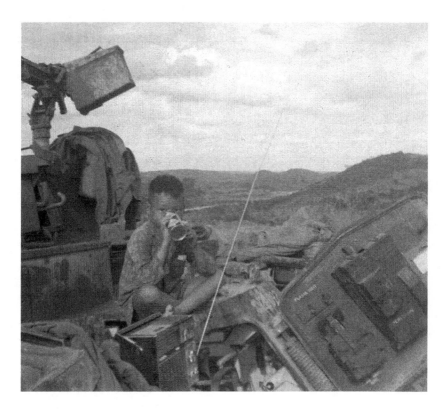

Lan makes himself comfortable on the Duster.

17

Coming Home

March 6, 1969, the day I came "back to the world."

The difference between Pacific time in California and Vietnam is fourteen hours. When it is 10 a.m. in California, it will take fourteen hours before it is 10 a.m. the same day in Vietnam. My return flight was going to take about twenty-two hours. I remember thinking I was getting to live some of that day over, even if I were only on an airplane; at least I wouldn't be in Vietnam.

On March 4, I was with my crew on OP Ben at Camp Rockpile when I got a call from the base camp on the lima-lima. The land line was a hand-generated telephone that actually had wires running all the way from the base camp up the hill to our bunker, about a mile and a half away. The caller said, "Blaylock, pack your shit and be at headquarters battery tomorrow at 0900."

That call was the foundation for celebration. I grabbed a packet of cherry Kool-Aid my folks had sent. I mixed it up in our drinking water and celebrated with the crew by sipping a canteen cup of warm Kool-Aid and talking about memories of "Back in the World." We drank warm Kool-Aid because everything is warm in Vietnam. I was packed and ready to go the next morning at

0600 when we left the OP for our daily mine sweep of the road. Fortunately, the sweep went smoothly and without any delay. The crew dropped me off in front of headquarters battery at about 0825 and waited there with me until the convoy pulled out. We said our joyful, but sad goodbyes and all promised to write each other.

I felt conflicted about leaving. I wanted to stay, not abandon my best buddies in that hell of a shit-hole place, Vietnam. On the other hand, I was going home, which had been the one single goal and focus of conversation for the entire year. Dennis and Len had arrived with me, but they had accepted the army's offer to extend their time in Vietnam by approximately three months in exchange for 150 days off their active duty commitment. I got in the back of a deuce-and-a-half, and gave the guys a wave as the convoy headed out to Dong Ha.

When I got to battalion headquarters in Dong Ha, I received orders to go to Cam Ranh Bay, and then on to the Seattle-Tacoma airport, and finally to Fort Lewis for processing and return to stateside, "the World." At Dong Ha, I walked up the loading ramp of a C-130 and sat in a web sling seat hanging from the walls of the airplane.

In Cam Ranh Bay, while waiting for my next flight home, I watched a steady stream of "Cherries" arriving. They wore clean fatigues and stiff-billed ball caps. As I looked at them, I thought how much they looked out of place. They had an unmistakable look of confusion and fear. They continuously looked around, searching their environment for whatever they thought would bring them comfort. I found myself almost grinning as they passed by. I didn't say anything to any of them. What could I say? Nothing, except think, "You poor SOBs don't have a clue. Good luck."

The flight from Cam Ranh Bay to Seattle-Tacoma utilized a commercial airliner, duplicating my original in-bound transport on a Boeing 707. Most of us returning GIs were still dirty because we had come directly from our units in the field. It was loud inside the plane for the first couple of hours, and then it turned quiet and somber. I don't know if it was that we were tired or if it was a feeling of remorse, guilt, or maybe even a fear of what we faced ahead. Had the world changed or had we? I guess we would know in a few hours. En route from Cam Ranh Bay, Vietnam, to Seattle, Washington, we made the obligatory stop in Japan to refuel the plane. It took just thirty minutes, and the plane parked out on the ramp, away from the terminal. Just like the trip over, they told us to say seated because we would not be getting off.

I remember thinking that the stewardesses appeared old. Had my perceptions changed? Maybe they were old, maybe twice my age, but they were nice. I imagine that most of the airline flight crews liked the military flight assignments because, as passengers, we weren't demanding. We were just glad to be sitting in that jet airplane on our way home. No alcohol was served, just soda and juice, and I should have had clear thoughts about the future. I replayed the Box Tops' popular song in my mind, "Gimme a Ticket."

Everyone in Vietnam sang that song, especially when we were getting short. While waiting to takeoff, someone started a song by the Animals, and then we all sang the refrain together: "We got to get out of this place if it's the last thing we ever do."

Arriving in Ft. Lewis, Washington, still dirty and in jungle fatigues, muddy boots, and sweat, I stood in line. When I reached the front of the line, I was measured and fitted for a new class-A-uniform. I took a hot shower and ate a cooked-to-order steak and potato dinner while my new uniform was being tailor-made. After that, I received my next orders, ones that included a thirty-day leave.

MOM AND DAD MET ME AT THE Los Angeles Airport.

Mom grabbed me first, hugged, and kissed me while Dad stood next to us patiently waiting his turn. His arms came around me and pulled me close by pulling hard against my back. Chest-to-chest and cheek-to-cheek, it was a long, strong hug, pushing the metal pins on the inside of my new uniform medals into my chest. It was a solid feeling of love and warmth. He said, "I'm glad you're home."

I remember the handshake and then that hug. He shook my hand with his strong right hand that felt as strong as steel, yet at the same time gentle.

My parents dropped me off at the apartment building, where Bonnie was living. It was an apartment on the ground floor of a two-story apartment complex. The front door was a sliding-glass patio door, and there were curtains covering it. I could hear the sound of a vacuum running when I knocked on the door. I stood at attention in my new tailored uniform. The curtains pulled back, and there was Bonnie. She screamed, then let go of the curtains as she started to turn away in a panic. She came back to the door, opened it, and jumped into my arms.

I had been home almost a week when we visited my parents, and my mom gave me a letter from Vietnam, addressed to me in care of my parents' address. It came to them from one of the marines that I had been with on OP Ben when I left. Several weeks before I left Nam, there was a squad of marines stationed with us on OP Ben. Several of them had become fairly close to our squad, spending a lot of time together playing cards, listening to AFBN, talking about women, and just general "BS."

I opened the letter from the marine. I read it quietly to myself, broke down, and started to cry. He told me that the day after I left Vietnam, their squad had been sent out on a search and destroy mission. They had been in the bush three days when they were caught in an ambush. He and one other marine were the only survivors of the squad. He was writing me from the hospital where he was being treated for leg wounds from shrapnel. He would be OK, he said, and would be returning to his unit in a week or so.

"They're dead! They're all fucking dead!" I said aloud as tears filled my eyes, blurring my vision.

Then, I started thinking to myself, "Why did I come home, and they didn't? I should have died there with them!"

TEARS FLOWED FROM MY EYES. I tried to wash them clean as the dust was caking up in corners. The chopper was whirling up so much of the damn red dirt from the freshly cleared LZ that it looked as if we were bleeding from our eyes. The noise was all around, and it consumed us along with the hurricane winds below the rotor blades. Blood and loose bandages were blowing out the open doors. Still we were able to get the wounded aboard and give them a thumbs-up as the dust-off rose skyward, taking them to a better place.

"Bill? Bill, are you OK?" Dad asked, standing a short, but reasonably safe distance away.

I RETURNED TO REALITY. My family sat there in the living room, Bonnie, Mom, and Dad, just looking at me with shocked expressions on their faces. Maybe they were shocked at my language or my sudden outburst in reaction to the letter. Maybe they were engaged with some fear of their own, seeing me suddenly tense-up in rage or sensing I had just zoned out for a bit. Maybe they were afraid I was losing it. If so, they would have been right. I went to the kitchen to get some water; Dad followed me and just stood with me, his hand on my shoulder. Nonetheless, after that, no one said a thing. I was left alone, alone to try to hold back my tears, my rage, and my guilt. That was the last time, until nearly forty years later, that I talked about Vietnam. I never answered his letter. I could not bring myself to face Vietnam again. I feel like such an ass for not answering him. He needed my support, and I failed him.

AFTER RETURNING HOME FROM VIETNAM, I still had another six months left in the army to complete my two-year draft obligation. While in Nam, I made plans about what I would do when I got home, but regrettably, the plans were not to be. In retrospect, my plans were selfish, but I thought that Bonnie and I would make love for two or three days straight, buy a new 1969 Chevy Nova, and I would enroll in flight training. Although I thought that those were reasonable intentions, they were not what Bonnie had been thinking about; she had her own agenda. She was in school and working a job. They were foremost on her mind, and she thought that when I got home, I would be helping with the responsibilities of income and household. I guess we were probably both disappointed about our plans for my return. When I got my orders to report to Fort Bliss, Texas, I had no idea where it was, except that it was in Texas, and I had never heard of it. While home, I looked it up on a map. Two days before having to report to duty, Bonnie and I packed up her light green Dodge Valiant and headed east on Interstate 10, taking us to El Paso and Fort Bliss. The terrain along the southern borders of New Mexico and Texas are mostly level compared to the Central Highlands of Vietnam, and that was just fine with me.

A few days after arriving at Fort Bliss, I looked up Cuba, my friend in Vietnam. Cuba returned to "the World" in August, 1968 and stationed at Fort Bliss until he completed his enlistment. In Nam, he had been my sergeant, leader, instructor, mentor, and friend. When I got to his barracks, I was surprised to see that it seemed to be segregated. I was stopped at the door and asked who I was and what I wanted. I asked if Cuba was there. I was told to wait where I was. A short while later Cuba came out. I was fully expecting a joyous reunion, but it was not to be.

To my sad awakening we were back in the real world—he in his and me in mine. When I saw Cuba approaching from within the hallway, I started toward him; he waved, gesturing me to stop. I waited for him to arrive. A moment later we shook hands and gave the usual greeting, "Hey man, how ya doin'?" Cuba said. "How 'bout we talk out here?" pointing down at the stairs to the barrack. So we sat down. We visited on the steps of his barracks for a while, but it was not the reunion I had wanted or was hoping for.

"What ya been doing since you got back," I asked. "Did you enjoy your time at home before coming here?"

"Oh yeah, it was good. Momma made me some cook'n, and it was good," putting extra emphasis and stretching out the O sound in good. "I got to see my old friends from my neighborhood; yeah it was good. How 'bout you?"

"Yeah, me too, it wasn't what I expected, but I guess I don't really know what I expected, but I'm back now, so it's all right." I said.

"Yeah," Cuba affirmed.

There was silence. Neither of us knew what to say next. I don't know who spoke first, but somehow we ended the visit saying, "Check ya later."

"Yeah, check ya later man."

I stood up from the step and walked back to my office. That is the last time I saw or spoke to Cuba.

Although I never thought we had solved the world's problems with our talking and getting to know each other in Nam, I was sure that we did have a special place in our hearts for each other. I left that day feeling disappointed in Cuba and how he had changed. Looking back, not just Cuba had changed. It was both of us, and our environments. It has taken me a long time to understand that in Nam we had to depend on each other, and did; but once back home, we had different people to be responsible to and to depend upon. Fair or not, that is the way it has been for a long time, unfortunately. It is a disappointment that makes me feel so very sorry and sad.

Although neither Cuba nor I physically died in Vietnam, our friendship did die there. It became another loss, leaving a constant emptiness in my soul. Our friendship would have not been possible if it were not for the war. Maybe, since it was born there, it had to die there also. I will never know the answer, but maybe there in that place, Vietnam, our friendship flourished in the only environment it could. In my heart, I could not let myself believe that.

MY TIME AT FORT BLISS WAS FAIRLY EASY and uneventful. Fort Bliss was a large facility; it had to be to allow for an artillery range. The base was also home to an airport named Biggs Field. Since it had runways long enough to accommodate large aircraft, I presumed it had been for training during the Second World War. There was a flying club on base, and I was able to take a few lessons in a Piper Cherokee 140 and rent the plane to solo a couple of times. I loved the feeling of flying. Although when with an instructor, I always felt anxious. There was always the feeling, once in the air, I needed to use the bathroom. I hated it. It seemed that nearly every time I flew I wouldn't be up but just a few minutes after take-off, when I would feel the urge. Of course, I couldn't take the time to go back, land, and pee, so I had to resist the urge. However, it did make for a few fast final landing approaches in an effort to get to the terminal as fast as possible.

For a short time, approximately two weeks after arriving at Fort Bliss, I was assigned to guard duty. I watched over army inmates while they worked outside the brig. After that, I went to headquarters battery to take on a supply clerk position and only worked Monday through Friday. I was in charge of expendable supplies. Expendable supplies are items that are not generally accounted for, such as cleaning supplies, brushes and brooms, paint, small hand tools, hammers, picks, shovels, and pocketknives. I included pocketknife in the list because it was a popular item, and I gave one to everybody who wanted one.

I took a pickup truck to the base warehouse to shop, where I bought supplies that would outfit the four batteries. My army credit card had my battalion's account number, and it would allow me to pay the warehouse. I managed my allocated funds accurately and stayed within my allotted budget most of the time, occasionally requesting extra allotments. I worked by myself, and I had my own small office. My office door split in half, top and bottom, creating a writing self on the bottom portion, but, more often, visitors just used the shelf. On one occasion, circumstances evolved around my supply clerk position to bring me a memorable bit of enjoyment and pride, especially because events circumvented the usual chain of command.

Our base was scheduled for a review by the inspector general. Such inspections are accompanied by a long list of silly, extraneous, nonsense rules requiring certain supplies and equipment be in proper order. One particular requirement was that each of the four batteries of the battalion store a particular amount of paint in specific colors in their respective battery lockers, a storage shed accessible to each battery. As the headquarters battery supply clerk, my job was to get the paint and similar types of items for the batteries when they requested it. Just hours before the scheduled inspection, the battalion commander, a colonel, came in the office asking for me specifically by name, calling out, "Specialist Blaylock!"

I thought to myself, "Oh shit, what did I do." Of course, I immediately responded to his call, "Yes Sir!"

The colonel's action was incredibly out of order. Normally he would have told a lower ranking officer, who would have told the warrant officer, who would have either told me. Or he would have had yet another sergeant tell me to make sure the order was carried out. Instead, the colonel reached up. Putting his hand on my shoulder, he started walking me outside to where the lockers were located. He asked if I thought that I could make sure that each locker had its respective paint and supply requirements inside it before the inspection. I assured him that I could make it happen. As we re-entered the office where my two ranking sergeants and a warrant officer were on duty at their desks, the colonel shook my hand and said, "Thank you!" The astonishment on their faces delighted me.

The two sergeants, one in particular, did not like me. I didn't like him either. I thought he was a kiss ass. We had all been in Vietnam, so perhaps we were having PTSD problems, or we simply didn't get along, but the dislike was mutual. I considered that perhaps the colonel didn't like them either, and he intentionally snubbed them by coming to me personally. But I could clearly see their red faces and tight jaws, evidence of their envy and chagrin. To ice the cake, the colonel returned later that afternoon after the inspection to thank me for my excellent work—a double snub to my two outranking sergeants!

My wife and I rented a small duplex apartment off base. Fort Bliss is located near El Paso, Texas, along the Mexico border. Bonnie and I had married while I was home on Christmas leave, and then I went to Vietnam for a year. So this was our first time to set up housekeeping and live together for more than a couple of weeks. We married young and soon after meeting. Our little one-bedroom duplex apartment was sufficient for the two of us. I was happy there. I went to work each day, and she stayed home. It was basic, and we didn't have much money, but it was all we needed.

The exterior of the duplex needed painting, so for partial payment of one month's rent, I painted the whole building. The color on the can was marked goldenrod, but I think it was closer to baby-poop yellow. While painting, I developed a blister on the forefinger of my right hand. I lanced it with my pocketknife and went on painting. Within days, my finger had swollen larger than my thumb, so I went to sick call at the base hospital. The attending army doctor had a medic stand by to help hold my hand still while he lanced my finger to drain the pus and then pack a long narrow strip of gauze bandage into the fresh wound he had just created. I wish he had given me anesthetic. I had to return every day for a repeat performance of this routine for about five days until my finger finally stopped oozing and didn't need to be packed with gauze anymore. Forty years later, I still have a scar on my finger to remind me.

El Paso was not home for me, but it was a whole hell of a lot better than Vietnam. They mowed the grass in El Paso. Trees were colorful, not the deep, dark-dark green of rotting Vietnamese vegetation. El Paso had hills and mountains, far enough away from my home to make it seem flat to me. Paved streets did not throw dirt and dust into the air when a vehicle passed by. Of course, we had our dust and dirt, but it was not red. El Paso was arid; there was humidity, but it wasn't wet all the time like Vietnam. The air was dry enough that everything would dry within a reasonable amount of time if left out.

Most weekends included a trip across the border to Juarez, Mexico for some sightseeing, shopping, entertainment, and cheap booze. Juarez had constructed a new stadium for dog racing. We made friends with another young couple who lived about two blocks away. They had a baby boy, less than a year old. I enjoyed holding and playing with him. We would occasionally all get together and travel south. At the dog races, a bell would ring and starting-gate doors would open to release the greyhounds. A fake rabbit mounted on a rail at the inside edge would lead the dogs around the track. At the finish line, the fake rabbit retracted into its receiver, and the dog handlers collected the dogs. It was fun to watch, a cheap source of evening entertainment.

When we got home from an evening with our friends, Bonnie complained that all I did all night was play with the baby. I presumed she was jealous. Before getting married, we had decided that we should not have any kids until Bonnie was finished with college, which turned out to be our best decision. We did not argue or fight much, but she complained that I shut her out and didn't talk to her. Almost every day when I got home, I just wanted to sit in a chair in the corner and watch TV shows like, Marcus Welby MD, Hee Haw, the Beverly Hillbillies, and Mission Impossible.

Although I worked with a fort full of GIs who had returned from Vietnam, none of us talked about it. Back then nearly everyone watched the evening news that was filled with stories of losses and body counts of American soldiers and marines. Television, newspapers, and magazines all told about peace marches, demonstrations, and clashes with police as anti-war protestors dominated the news. We viewed pictures of protestors holding signs that called us "baby killers" and "warmongers." We were disgraced and disrespected by our country, friends, and even some of our families. I think that we—at least I— just didn't want to remember. Perhaps, since it seemed that we had returned in shame, none of us wanted to confront our obvious defeat, nor did I want to return to Vietnam in my memories or conversations.

Bonnie applied and was accepted to San Jose State College, so she left for the start of school in September about three weeks before my discharge. I figured that when I returned I would get a job and go to school using my GI Bill benefits to become a commercial pilot. When I discharged, I returned to Covina to visit with my parents for a couple of days before going north to San Jose where Bonnie's father had purchased a small home for us to rent from him. Bonnie's sister and brother-in-law already lived next door.

I enrolled in junior college under the GI Bill, which gave me extra money each month to use for education. I declared aviation as my major. Flight time was expensive. The instructor got $12 per hour. The aircraft cost $18 per hour plus fuel, which was sold at about $1.50 per gallon. The plane burned three and a half gallons per hour. Even with the GI bill giving me about $100 per month, I couldn't get a private pilot license, let alone a commercial license which required several hundred hours of instruction and solo flights. Besides, I already had more than sixty hours logged, and I wasn't ready to take my FAA check ride. It seemed to me that most pilots were getting their license after about forty-five hours. My decision was clear: quit and try something else. I felt like a failure for quitting flying, but my wife perceived my failure as not being able to keep and maintain a steady job.

I had worked at two gas stations, Montgomery Wards selling shoes, Sears in the men's clothing department, and two airlines as a ramp serviceman loading and unloading luggage on airplanes. I sold cars and was a security guard. In the two years after my discharge from the army, September 1969 until September 1971, I worked at nine different jobs. Some employers fired me, but more often I quit. I tended to be argumentative with fellow employees and supervisors and, I just didn't give a crap. Everything and everybody made me mad. One time, when working at one of the gas station jobs, I arrived to work four minutes late. The boss told me, "You need to be here at work early and ready to start on time."

I said, "I was only four minutes late; that's no big deal."

"Yes, it is a big deal. You're late every time."

"Fine then, I won't be late anymore, I quit!"

No matter what I did, there was some jerk telling me what to do and how to do it. In Vietnam, nobody told me what to do; we just did what we needed, and got the job done. A couple of times I told a boss, "This is a bunch of bullshit, I quit." Then I'd walk out.

I should have realized something was not right. I never would have reacted like that before going in the army.

I flinched and reacted every time there was a loud or sudden noise. I was always on the ready, hyper-vigilant. Many times during the night, I would wake up yelling, "oncoming," or "shot out." I would be out of bed trying to take cover on the floor before I realized where I was. I always needed to know what was behind me. At restaurants and public places, I needed to sit in a corner or with my back to a wall. I had to know my surroundings and environment and still do to this very day. I could not relax in large groups of people. I was constantly looking around trying to find an exit. I became rapidly anxious and irritable in crowded places. My behavior became frustrating for my wife, making her irritable. In turn, that would upset me even more.

At church one Sunday, when I refused to get trapped between people and wanted to be on the end of the pew near the back of the church for a quick exit, Bonnie got upset and had to go outside to cool down. Outside we got into an argument. She told me, "This is church. There isn't anything in there to be afraid of."

"I'm not afraid of anything. I just don't like being squeezed between people and not able to move if I have to!"

She constantly complained and asked, "Why can't you keep a job?" That would be followed by another inquiry: "Why don't you like people anymore? Why do we always have to sit at a corner table or against the wall? Can't we just sit where there is an available table?"

"Because they are all a bunch of assholes," I would often reply. Sometimes I just wished I were dead! If she wanted to go to a group function, I told her to go without me, so I could stay home alone. I was happier that way, not having to deal with a bunch of opinionated, mocking, demoralizing, duplicitous, phony people.

She participated in the college choir. The choir had a picnic at a local city park close to the campus, and choir members were to bring a date or guest. The choir had nearly seventy members. If each brought a guest, that would be nearly 140 people. They would be people I didn't know, and besides, I told myself, I had seen the choir before. I knew that there would not be many *real men* there. I figured that those choir guys were all queer anyway. I couldn't be there, crowded around all those people and strangers, and then watch that.

"It's not for me!" I said. "You can go if you want, but leave me out."

She did go by herself, and that would not be the last event she attended alone. I always felt like I was being judged, and I did not want to be around people.

My parents repeatedly asked in phone calls if I was all right and why was I making all those job changes. I was in denial to them and to myself. I told my parents that I was fine and was only changing jobs to make more money. I told them that I had not been having any bad dreams or thinking about Vietnam, although I knew that was not true.

Meanwhile, I did think about Cuba and how our friendship ended. I thought about Leonard, Dennis, and all the other guys.

IN SEPTEMBER 1971, I ACCEPTED a position with the San Jose Police Department. A federal program that would help minorities, underprivileged, and veterans funded the department. As a veteran, I qualified for the program and was hired. I enjoyed the job and quickly became interested in law enforcement as a career. My duties included inspection and removal of abandoned vehicles and serving subpoenas. I began to develop a sense of self-respect and worth. Plus having a badge, even though it was engraved "Police Cadet," established a high level of pride and responsibility. I was finally doing something of importance. I got to drive around in both marked and unmarked police vehicles. I enrolled in law enforcement classes at San Jose City College and attended classes that the police department provided. I held that job for almost two years until the program for police cadets ended in July 1973.

Just three short months after starting my new job with the San Jose Police Department, Dad contracted pancreatic cancer and was admitted to the VA Hospital in Long Beach. He had multiple conditions of heart disease, yellow jaundice, and pancreatic cancer. Dad had been in the hospital about two weeks. The doctors had operated on his pancreas. Shortly after coming out of surgery, he went into a coma. I flew down on my days off, and thankfully, the department was generous allowing me to take extra time off. I arrived at the hospital the second weekend, and Dad had been comatose for about two hours. Both Mom and I stayed at the hospital the whole weekend. About three hours before I returned to San Jose, Dad woke from his coma. He was groggy, but coherent and smiling to see us. We both talked and told him how worried we were and how much we loved him. I was able to return to work knowing Dad was OK.

When I got home from the airport, Bonnie told me Mom had called and that I should call her back. I picked up the phone and called the number at the hospital. Mom's voice was soft, almost difficult to hear, with a slight pause, she said, "Bill, your father died a few minutes after you left the hospital."

Hanging up the phone, and standing with my back to the wall, I slid down to the floor and remained there in the fetal position for a half hour, quietly weeping.

December 7, 1971, Dad died in the VA Hospital, in Long Beach, California. Mom survived him by twenty-six more years before her own passing on November 17, 1997.

In April 1973, Bonnie and I separated and filed for divorce, citing irreconcilable differences. After less than six years of marriage, one of which I was in Vietnam, our marriage was over. The Superior Court of Santa Clara County granted our divorce in late September that same year. When the divorce was final, I felt relief, free of my anxiety and its binds. I wasn't responsible to anyone, particularly a wife. I didn't have to act or pretend like I cared, not to her, nor to anyone else. I could do as I pleased. What a relief! Later I would learn that one of the PTSD symptoms is numbing to personal relationships, and I was doing a good job of shutting people out.

"Hey Tim, can I stay at your place a while?"

18

Moving On

When people asked me about Vietnam, I told them about the dark-night sky with all the bright stars. I told about buying a bottle of Gook rum from Vietnamese people at the roadside. We always had to check the bottle to make sure there was no ground glass in it. After one mine sweep, we bought a bottle and passed it around in the bunker later that day. We told Len he could finish it, so he tipped it back and drank it to the bottom. He abruptly turned toward the door and passed out, falling on the steps, face first.

I told them about using a P-38 can-opener. I told people about how delightful it was to get a care package from my parents with stale homemade cookies and Kool-Aid. Kook-Aid was the only thing that made the stinking muddy river water taste halfway decent. Every soldier and grunt in Vietnam wanted it. When someone got a care package from home, it was, greatly appreciated.

I told them about the time that I thought Christ was making his second coming while I was on guard duty on OP Ben. I saw a pure white light radiating from the horizon in the east. I stared at it for what seemed to be thirty minutes before I finally saw the brilliant white dome of the moon crest over the eastern mountains.

I told people about the time I shot Leonard in his left forearm with a pellet pistol that my wife had sent me to shoot rats inside our bunker.

I told about leeches in the water and the enormous tan-colored spiders that were so big I could hear their bones break when I stepped on them. I told about showering in the monsoon rains. There was the dirt. The filthy, stinking red dirt—it was everywhere, on and in everything. How could a jungle grow so green in red dirt?

I told about returning from a morning mine sweep along Highway 9 and spotting the wild boar with her piglets. I didn't tell about the massacre; I just said we had some barbecued wild pork that night.

It would be many years before making the connection between my attitude toward people, emotional numbing, and reoccurring nightmares to having post-traumatic stress disorder.

After Bonnie and I separated, I lived with my best friend, Tim. After my position with San Jose police ended in July 1973, I worked for Trans World Airlines as a ramp serviceman. My duties ranged from cleaning aircraft after passengers disembarked, to loading and unloading baggage and freight from aircraft. It wasn't an exciting job, but it was a fairly good paying one with medical benefits plus discounted travel. The only drawback was the long forty-five minute commute each way, to San Francisco International Airport.

Tim and I lived in an apartment in San Jose. Ours was the front unit of a triplex: one apartment downstairs in front, one on the side, and one accessible upstairs in back. One early summer evening in May, Tim and I had the stereo playing a Deep Purple album when we heard a knock on the door. Tim answered it to see a man wearing a cowboy hat, t-shirt, jeans, and western boots. He introduced himself, "I'm your neighbor; Manuel Celaya, and I've got to tell you that the loud radio in the morning is waking me up an hour before I need to get up, and I'd really appreciate it if you'd turn it down."

Tim was then and still is, according to his wife Melody, an unusually heavy sleeper who was not awakened by a mere radio coming on. He had to turn up the volume of the radio to its maximum, and then it would play for several minutes before he would respond to it. As it turned out, Tim's window faced the direction of Manuel's apartment, and the sound carried across the seventy feet of unobstructed lawn between the two apartments. Tim apologized for the loud radio, and Manuel invited us over to his house to have a beer and meet his wife Alice and his daughter Gina.

It was a comfortably warm evening in May. We sat in lawn chairs, visiting and enjoying that cold beer. Tim and I hadn't been there very long when a pretty young woman rode up on her bicycle. Alice introduced her to us as her sister, Betty. Betty was in her early twenties with a pleasant smile. She had beautiful, long, wavy, reddish-brown hair. The wavy curls of her hair came down over her shoulders and down her back to just above her shoulder blades.

Betty remembers that at one point in the evening I got down on the ground to show off by performing several one-arm pushups. What a dope I was, but apparently it worked. We fell in love and got married the following year.

I was able to get discounted tickets to Hawaii for our honeymoon. Airline employees could purchase flights for the price of the tax on the full fare cost of the ticket. We flew standby, which got us bumped off every flight for the next day and a half. Nearly thirty hours passed until there was a flight with two seats available. In spite of the delays, we were two young newlyweds on honeymoon in Hawaii.

While we enjoyed ourselves on the island, the airline stewardess's union went on strike and stayed out three days. After a strike, all unionized laborers were required to report to work within forty-eight hours, and I was in that category of employment. I told myself, "Well, what the hell, man, I am in Hawaii on my honeymoon." I still had three days left of my scheduled vacation. Since I was on an approved vacation, I assumed there was no need to return within the forty-eight hour report window. In addition, I didn't see any need to worry Betty about the return-to-work rule. I figured my absence was approved, and all was well. I would just keep the issue to myself.

When I reported to work after returning from Hawaii, it was the third day after the return to work call. I received a letter saying I had violated the company-union agreement to return to work within forty-eight hours after a strike settlement. That pissed me off, so I told them what I thought of their stupid-assed, company-union agreements, and I stomped out.

At the time, Tim was working as a machinist at a shop in Redwood City. Since I had taken a couple of semesters of machine shop in high school, he was able to get me a job with his employer. I ran a lathe, cutting steel production parts for a contract the shop had. That lasted only two months until I got laid off due to lack of work.

In April 1974, my now brother-in-law, Manuel, a truck driver, helped me get a position where he worked so I could learn to drive a truck. I got my class-one commercial driver's license and became a big-rig driver. That lasted until August the same year until the company suffered a work shortage. Since I was the newest employee, I was the first to be let go.

Over the next ten months, I worked as a security guard with two different outfits before being called back to the truck-driving job for a short-term summer driving position in 1975. Employers didn't do background checks much in those days. When a potential employee interviewed well, the employer trusted his own judgment. In addition, despite the unpopularity of the war, employers seemed to be happy to hire a veteran. I have always been able to interview and communicate well with people, and that got me a job each time I needed one.

When the trucking job ended that summer, I was able to get another driving job that lasted until I quit to take a position with the San Francisco Airport Police. I was happy there and stayed from October 1975 to February 1980 when I got the itch to move on and try something else.

Jobs came and went. In the forty-two years after my military discharge, I held thirty-six jobs. I drove trucks, worked as a security guard, and for nine of those forty years worked as a correctional officer.

I sold cars and solar water heaters. I was in partnership with a friend in a janitorial business cleaning restaurant kitchens. I owned two businesses. I bought a three-axle truck tractor, contracting as a sub-hauler of cryogenics, liquid oxygen, nitrogen, and argon. Then I owned a coffee house. Betty and I worked together, had fun and met a lot of people, but it was difficult running a business, and we didn't make any money.

I WONDER WHAT LEONARD, DENNIS, and Cuba are doing. I hope they're OK!

19

Influences of PTSD

Sometime in early 2011, I pondered how PTSD has affected me and what kind of father have I been. I believe I have been a good father to my kids. I am sure, however, I was overly protective when they were young and especially teen-aged. I ensured I knew where they were and with whom at all times. My wife says that I am more than over protective; I was strict. Sometimes those two actions overlap.

My daughter Tiffany, kind in her response, said that if I had, in fact, been overprotective, she assumed that was the way all fathers were. She did say, however, that I was rash without reason. She concluded I simply didn't know what to do with a teenage daughter who was too old to take out for donuts or a milkshake as a way of building our father-daughter relationship. She followed up, saying: "I know you to be a very caring father, one whom I could count on to help me or any of my friends."

I am guarded with my feelings; I feel protected that way. I am afraid to let go of emotional control and have worked hard to protect myself.

Psychiatrists call it "emotional numbing." Giving my whole self would make me vulnerable, exposed, and weakened to someone or to the pain of losing the relationship. I felt it better not to let myself become vulnerable; otherwise, it would reveal my inner self and I could expose myself to pain.

I PREFER TO KEEP MYSELF ISOLATED. I like my alone time. I am uncomfortable both in crowds and in small groups of people.

One evening Betty and I accepted an invitation to a friend's home. We four couples visited in the kitchen; the wives chatted at one end of the kitchen island, the men on the other. If you were to ask, all would say they were having a marvellous time, intent on fellowship. However, I found myself weary of the conversation and tired of playing nice. I headed to the bathroom, but on the way passed a comfortable living room. In the corner by the window sat a rocking chair with a soft, brightly colored cushion.

I sat down in the rocker and instantly began to feel better. The warm evening sun filtered through the window, bringing a smile to my face. I listened to the frivolous, inconsequential conversation in the next room while I enjoyed being alone. Then I tensed.

I heard Betty's voice. "Where's Bill?" I sat in silence and then heard her again, saying, "Maybe he went outside. I'll check."

I watched as she walked past the room where I sat, saw her open the front door, and take one or two steps outside, calling, "Bill...Bill, are you out here?"

I knew I should answer, but I did not. Betty closed the door and turned to go back to the kitchen when she saw me sitting in the rocker. "Why didn't you answer me?"

Her frustration showed in her face and voice. I cannot explain why I needed to escape. I cannot explain why I didn't answer. I grimaced and shrugged my shoulders in reply. Betty returned to the kitchen, leaving me where I sat. Soon she made excuses to the others about my being tired and that she needed to get me home.

TRAFFIC IS A SOURCE OF FRUSTRATION for many people, not just those of us with PTSD. However, for me, it is a significant problem. Just like being in a crowd of people, I get anxious and aggravated when in congestion. I don't have to be the one driving either. Even as a passenger, I become nervous and fidgety when riding in the car. My wife says that my hands and fingers are constantly moving and twitching. I like cars, but maybe it is because of the confinement of my surroundings and not the traffic alone. I wouldn't be surprised to find out that the phrase "road rage" was coined by a veteran with PTSD.

There are traffic laws and rules of the road. Why can't people follow them? Damn! It is provoking to pull up to an intersection only to have the stupid asshole across the street make a left turn in front of me without signaling. Man, that pisses me off! I mean how lazy does a person have to be to not exercise the little finger on their left hand to activate the turn signal switch—one finger, up or down. Also, if you don't want to drive the posted speed limit, pull over. Let the rest of us pass, and you can continue your leisurely stroll after we go by.

THAT BRINGS UP ANOTHER DRIVING problem, well not actually driving, but parking. Most vehicles are about six-feet wide or less. Traffic lanes are ten feet wide, and parking spaces are usually eight feet wide. I can't understand why drivers can't steer their vehicles into the approximate center of a parking space, allowing the adjacent space its full availability. For some people, parking must be like the movie *Star Wars*. It is easier to go to the dark side. Doing wrong must have a stronger force field.

On one occasion, I was unable to contain my frustration when my wife and I traveled to a weekend getaway in Lake Tahoe. We stopped at a local shopping mall. I parked within the allowed space, and we went browsing in the stores. When we returned, another vehicle parked too close to the drivers' side of our car. Less than one foot separated our vehicles, obviously not enough room for me to get in my car through the driver-side door. Betty was already sitting in the passenger seat when I got to my side of our car.

Anger built. My previous temptations to act out in such circumstances had been suppressed. Not today. I had to do something to this stupid asshole for being so inconsiderate and for being such a lousy driver. I squeezed in between our two vehicles, pressing my key up against the passenger door of that car. Then moving back to the rear of the car, I left a wonderfully deep scratch in the paint of that new vehicle. It stretched from the front passenger door through the second passenger door and onto the rear fender. All the while, my temper rising, I gave not a single thought to the correctness or incorrectness of my action. I wanted revenge and now felt justified. No forethought, just action!

"There you stupid ass," I thought to myself, feeling somewhat proud.

Just then I heard a voice say, "Hey, what do you think you're doing? That's my new car."

Oops, reality set in. Instantly, I knew I was wrong, but I still felt justified. We had a succinct dialogue about what a shitty driver he was and how incompetent he was at parking. Then he pointed to the vehicle on the other side of him, which was parked diagonally in a horizontal parking space. This is where he went to the dark side. He said, "Look at how they parked. What was I supposed to do?"

I said, "Well, you stupid SOB. You could have parked correctly or not parked there at all if there wasn't space to park correctly!"

I wore an olive, drab-green t-shirt, embroidered with a U.S. Army insignia on the chest pocket.

He asked, "Are you a veteran?"

"Yes."

He took the initiative to cool down the situation, saying, "I have a lot of respect for veterans, so let's not make me call the sheriff."

I agreed. I was wrong for keying his car. I gave him my insurance information; he backed out his vehicle so I could get into mine, and that was the last we saw of each other. Of course, Betty was perturbed with me. It ruined our whole weekend, and it would ruin others when she would remind me of the occurrence. I know that I shouldn't get that upset about traffic, parking, and the annoying inconveniences of life, but I cannot fully harness my rage and anxiety.

20

Flashbacks and Triggers

While stopped at a traffic light, I hear a sudden loud cracking noise to my left, the unmistakable crack of an AK-47. I turn to look when...*pssssssng*. I can hear and feel the wind of the bullet pass by my left ear. I know, without a doubt that one was meant for me. Someone is actually trying to kill me. "Shit! Fire, fire, fire! Snipers in the trees! Fire!"

Noise erupts everywhere—yelling and shooting!

Marines hit the ground, trying to take cover while returning fire at the same time. I see some of them attempting to advance toward the sniper's location.

"Cuba, come left," I yell into the microphone on my helmet.

As he swings the guns left, I fire the two 40-mm guns of my Duster: *boom, boom, boom, boom, boom* sounds rattle in rapid succession. Dennis and Leonard load the four-round clips of ammo into the magazines of the guns as fast as I fire them. I don't know exactly where that sniper is, but I'm going to put out as many rounds as it takes to get that SOB. Our rounds rip branches off trees. They break and fly to the ground as we penetrate the jungle with furious, high-explosive ordinance and projectiles!

THEN *HONK*. THE DRIVER BEHIND me sounds his horn. The light is green. Off I go. A flashback! Thank God, I was stopped at the light and not moving when that false reality hit me. Fortunately for me, most of my flashbacks have occurred at a time of the day when I wasn't in a situation that would cause critical injury to anyone or serious embarrassment to me. I don't want anyone to know I'm crazy!

Flashbacks are especially alarming and dangerous. During a flashback, I go back in time and actually re-live an incident in present time. I can see, hear, smell, and feel the moment of my particular trauma. My mind puts me physically in that time and place, and I conduct myself in response to it. It not only happens to me, it happens to other veterans who suffer with PTSD. Obviously, a flashback can pose danger, both to the suffering veteran and others nearby, especially if the flashback takes the vet to an experience of extreme violence with access to weapons. Even in cases where no bystanders are present to witness a flashback and be vulnerable to injury, the victim of a flashback returns to reality feeling ashamed and humiliated.

My flashbacks usually last only a few minutes, but for the rest of my day, I am exhausted and disoriented. I have trouble focusing on my duties, following instructions, and staying on task. Afterwards, I have the urge to drink, zone out and attempt anything to escape. That is how PTSD affects me.

I enjoy going to air shows, especially military air shows. I'm proud of my country and enjoy seeing its strength displayed. Many shows feature C-130 and Huey aircraft, but they don't seem to incite any flashbacks. Maybe it is because I know in advance that I will be seeing and hearing them, rather than just suddenly hearing them unexpectedly. In reflection, the quick and unexpected trigger is what seems to provoke my flashbacks.

Fireworks! Now they make for a big event. Even though I know I am watching a Fourth of July celebration, the excitement and visual effect of the explosions recreate a time in the past when those flashes and explosions were for real and had a deadly purpose. Watching the rocket trail of the firework as it goes toward the sky is fun for the other spectators, but what I see is the red trail of a tracer round going toward its target in an attempt to cause death and destruction, allowing me to adjust my direction of fire when shooting at night.

I went to Hawaii in November of 1968 for an army-sanctioned period of rest and relaxation. My wife and parents all met me there. I remember my wife and I lying on the bed in our hotel room, just relaxing. Our room was situated five floors up. The balcony sliding door was open. From the balcony, we enjoyed a view of the tops of the palm trees below, the beach and ocean on the left side. Still reposed and enjoying each other's company, I heard a *thump*.

"Shot out, incoming," I yelled while rolling to the floor.

Next I heard the explosion of an artillery shell, followed by rapid automatic and small arms fire. Quickly I realized I was looking outside at the beach and toward the city of Waikiki. My young wife just looked down at me lying on the floor. She contorted her face with a look of surprise and said, "What's the matter with you?"

Apparently in Hawaii, or at least back then, they would put on a fireworks show on the beach each week. Not being aware of the tradition, I mistook the fireworks for the so-vivid reality of life at my OP in Vietnam.

Now, I actually do enjoy watching fireworks. I am proud of America and watching a fireworks demonstration gives me a patriotic tear when put to music of the "Star Spangled Banner." Even today, my experience of "rockets' red glare and bombs bursting in air" causes me to reflect on what Francis Scott Key was seeing when he wrote a poem that later became the lyrics of our national anthem.

After all these years, I still have not been able to determine all the circumstances that specifically might trigger a flashback. However, the unexpected sound of a Huey helicopter or a C-130 plane does initiate flashbacks and memories of Vietnam. The Huey usually causes me to remember supplies being dropped and medical evacuations. Medevac, also known as "dust-off," is the most common and most disturbing of my memories. I am haunted by that incident on Highway 9, east of our location at the Rockpile where casualties were so gruesome. Those marines were pinned down, ambushed, taking fire from both sides of the road. It was our job to load up as many injured as we could get on the Duster and transport them for dust-off.

Sometimes during my day, tears will come to my eyes, and I just start to cry for no apparent reason. I am usually able to get to a private place, but occasionally no refuge is in sight. Then I feel the shame and embarrassment of feeling as if I am crazy or a pussy or both.

I have learned that seeing a small child can prompt a flashback. My mind will go back to Vietnam when I see a child, especially one barefoot and donning worn-out clothes. I find myself remembering the young Vietnamese boy, Lan, who was eight-years old when I knew him in 1969. I met Lan while our battery was providing security for a Seabee's unit working on the Song Cam Lo River. The River is located in the northern region of South Vietnam, and it runs parallel with Highway 9. My flashback will take me to a lush dark-green jungle area located in the mountainous region. I will remember how the green colors blanket the landscape except for areas where our bombing and bulldozers have scraped the jungle forestation away, exposing the red dirt. And my mind will take me along the Song Cam Lo River, where the water was never clean, never blue, but always dirty brown or red.

Holidays are triggers. Every year at Thanksgiving and Christmas, I remember those holidays in Vietnam. On

Thanksgiving 1968, we had already eaten some C-rations when a chopper flew overhead and dropped out a couple of containers used to keep food warm. They didn't want to land, dropping them from a brief, fifteen–foot hover. The containers included some sliced turkey, mashed potatoes, gravy, and vegetables. Of course, all foods mixed together from the drop, but we all partook of a warm turkey dinner, nonetheless. I'm sure there were plenty of other troops who did not get turkey that day, let alone warm turkey, so I was thankful.

Christmas always proves difficult. Even with family and friends around, I am still reminded of Christmas in Vietnam. It bothers me more now than it did immediately after I first returned from the war. For so long, I was able to suppress those thoughts and emotions. Today, they rise up and I reflect on a picture of me standing in front of the bunker with a decorated Christmas tree, sent by my folks. My parents were faithful about sending regular care packages. The Christmas package was extra special that year. It contained the tree, broken cookies, and Kool-Aid that would transform the river water into refreshment. "Thanks, Mom and Dad," I think.

Today I enjoy Christmas each year, even though my mind so often returns to the experiences of Southeast Asia. If anyone asks about my most memorable Christmas, I have to describe Christmas of 1968, entrenched with buddies in the forsaken jungle of Vietnam.

Finally, I have identified corrugated tin as another flashback trigger. Every time I see that stuff, I am reminded of the time that someone had procured a canned ham from the mess tent at Camp Rockpile. We sliced and cooked it on a big sheet of the tin. The corrugated tin was galvanized, so, looking back, we probably should not have eaten anything that had been cooked on it. We didn't know any better then. Besides, we all pretty much figured we were going to die there anyway, so what the hell. "Go ahead and enjoy while we can," we thought. When

I see or hear about corrugated tin, it makes me remember—
and laugh.

IN AUGUST 1988, MY FAMILY AND I went to Puerto
Vallarta, Mexico for vacation. We flew from San Francisco direct
to Puerto Vallarta. My wife had taken care of making all the
arrangements, and she said that we were going to a sunny beach
location in Mexico for our vacation. Great, that was fine with
me, and the kids should like it too. All I had to do was request
the vacation time off. I loved it when she took care of this stuff
because I would just get upset trying to make reservations and
schedules.

We went to the airport, got on the plane, and off we flew south
to Mexico. All was well. The plane we were on was a DC-10. On
this particular aircraft, the doors do not swing open from a hinge.
Instead, they open electrically by sliding up. Therefore, if you are
standing inside the airplane, looking toward the door, the first
thing visible is the ground, and your view gradually increases as
the door continues to open. Our seats were located just a couple
of rows back from the divider that separates first class from coach.
They were excellent seats on that large airplane.

When we landed in Puerto Vallarta, and the plane parked, I
could see the terminal through my right side window. Everyone
got up, started to retrieve their luggage and paraphernalia from
the overhead storage compartments, and proceed to move toward
the door to prepare for exit.

In Puerto Vallarta, the aircraft do not pull up to the terminal
to dock with a jetway. Instead, the aircraft park away from the
terminal, on the tarmac; a portable stairway rolls up to the plane,
and everyone disembarks down the stairs toward the terminal.

"Good afternoon ladies and gentlemen," the airline captain
announced. "The time here is 12:47 p.m. The temperature is 88

degrees, and the relative humidity is 81. Thank you for flying with us today."

I was about five feet away from the door, with two rows of people in front of me. A stewardess stood next to the door with her hand on the control lever. As soon as the door broke its seal, I felt warm, humid air rush in. It gripped me as if it were strangling my throat. As the door opened a couple of inches above the floor, I could see the black tarmac below, heat waves rising up from the asphalt. I felt a strange hesitation in my enthusiasm.

The hatch kept moving up. Suddenly, when the door was just two feet above the floor of the plane, I saw the green trees of the jungle. I started trying to step back, but the sergeant is pushing me and saying, "Come on, let's go, move out!"

I couldn't move; I was frozen. I am standing at the door of the Western Airlines Boeing 707 with my duffle bag slung over my shoulder, waiting my turn to go down the stairs to report for duty here in Cam Ranh Bay.

My feet are planted as if glued to the floor. My wife is standing there behind me pushing and saying, "Come on, Bill, let's go!"

Aside from my hesitation and the flashback, the rest of the vacation was terrific, and I could even accept the airline losing one of our suitcases for a day.

21

Sam and Friends

The personal computer allows me to go to a place in my home where I will not be disturbed. I can shut out the world by playing solitaire, Free Cell, or a war game. I can even write, which my psychiatrist tells me is an excellent therapy for getting out my thoughts and aggressions. The problem, my wife says, is that I also shut her out. I don't intentionally mean to shut her out of my life; it is just what happens when I go to my place for my secluded soul time. I am usually at peace there, even if I am in reflection of a different time and place, and yes, even if it is sometimes painful.

Out of this environment, about October of 1999, I decided to attempt looking up my old Vietnam buddies. It took me 30 years and the Internet to make the attempt, but I had been thinking of them often.

WHEN I FIRST ATTEMPTED TO CONTACT Cuba, Leonard, and Dennis, I used the Internet to get addresses all across the country for each one of them. I didn't get any hits for Cuba, and I have tried several times since. With about eight matches for Dennis, and six for Leonard, I composed a letter to send to them, inserting each of their names where appropriate. The letter went something like this:

> *Dear Dennis,*
>
> *Thirty years ago (1968) I served in Vietnam with a man named Dennis Ramsey. We were on a Duster in the First, 44th C battery located at the Rockpile.*
>
> *If you are the person I am looking for, please call or write to the phone number or address below. I think of you often, and I pray that you are happy and well.*
>
> *If this letter does not apply, I thank you for your time and please disregard.*
>
> *Sincerely,*
>
> *William (Bill) Blaylock*

Over the next two to three weeks, several of the letters seeking Dennis and Leonard were returned, marked undeliverable. A couple of people were kind enough to write back to say that they were not the person I was looking for, but they wished me luck in finding them. Then one morning when returning from the mailbox, I heard a message left on the telephone answering machine. I didn't make it to the phone in time to catch the caller before he hung up, but I immediately recognized the voice. It was Leonard. His message said, "Hey Billy, this is Leonard. I just read your letter. What a surprise! I have thought about you all these years and didn't think I would ever hear or see you again. Hey, sorry I missed ya. Take care. Bye."

Maybe you can imagine how I felt, but I want to tell you that it was an amazing feeling of joy and relief. I felt joy to have finally made contact with a person that had meant so much to me all those years ago. It was a relief to know that I had not lost another casualty to Vietnam.

I grabbed the phone and called him right back.

"Hello," his unmistakable voice answered.

"Leonard, this is Bill! Hi. How are you? Man, it's good to hear your voice."

"Billy-Boy, I'm sure glad I got your letter. I'm doin' good, and still workin' at the plant. How 'bout you?"

"Yeah, I'm doin' fine too." There was a pause in our conversation.

Leonard said; "Dennis and I had been in contact most of the time since we came back home, but...uh...last year...Dennis was killed in a welding accident!"

"Oh shit!"

"Another loss," I thought, feeling a pain in my heart, and as if I wanted to cry.

"He has a sister who I write to," Leonard said, "and I know she would like to hear from you, too."

"Yeah, sure, what's her address?"

As I copied down her address, I was happy to finally be talking to Leonard, but there was an uncomfortable pause in our conversation. I suppose that we weren't exactly sure what we wanted to say to each other.

"Well, OK, Len, write or call whenever you want. It's sure good to finally talk to you again, so I'll let you go for now. Bye."

"Yeah, OK, Billy. Bye."

Leonard and I continued to write and call over the next few years, and still do.

In 2004, my wife Betty and I were able to take a driving

vacation to visit our friends Russ and Sue in Indiana. We planned to make the trip up to Alpena, Michigan, to visit Leonard and his wife, Julie. It is difficult to explain the excitement and joy that Leonard and I both felt when we finally saw each other again after thirty-five years. What an awesome reunion we had. The reunion, I believe, was an affirmation of our past. It wasn't just a long nightmare; it was real, and we are the living proof. The bonds of our relationship are an amazing example of the true loyalty of two men, who, after over forty years, still have a respect and dedication unsurpassed by any other kind of relationship. Betty, Julie, Leonard, and I all had a wonderful time together. I hope we will do it again someday before it's too late.

Leonard and Dennis had stayed in touch for those years after Vietnam. Unfortunately, Dennis's passing was disturbing news for me. Although it was not funny, it struck me that I could imagine him building a still to brew some corn whisky. The Dennis I know—that would have made him a happy man.

I regret that I had not made the effort to be a better friend and to contact them sooner. Maybe Dennis would have still been alive so that I could tell him how I felt about our exceptional bond.

Leonard gave me the address of Dennis's sister, Brenda, and I have written to her several times as well. I have not written as often as I should, but it is comforting to receive her letters. She often expresses to me her feelings for Dennis and tells me of her brother's feelings for Leonard and me. Brenda wrote me a letter that talked about all of her family. It drew me in and made me feel a part of Dennis's family. Though they cannot hear me, I send them my thoughts, saying "Brenda, thanks for making me feel like family when you write. Dennis, you were a good person and buddy, and you're here in my heart, always. So long, Cefus. Peace."

IN 2006 WHILE AT A FRIEND'S gathering, I was talking to my friend, Sam Topps. I had met Sam about twenty years before and had seen him just twice since. He is married to Kathy, my wife's best friend from high school. Although we had not spent much time together, Sam had also served in Vietnam, and I trusted him. I considered him a friend. Sam continued to serve his country for many more years in the U.S. Army and Army Reserve. Sam retired from the United States Army Reserve with the highest rank for a non-commissioned officer, sergeant major.

He told me about his recent experiences with the Veterans Administration, both good and bad.

Sam asked about my sleep patterns and if my sleep is interrupted by getting up to walk around the house to check the perimeter, which means to check that doors and windows are shut and locked and to look around outside to make sure things are in their proper place. He asked about recurring dreams and flashbacks. Sam made me realize that I wasn't the only one who did that.

"You've got it, man. You've got PTSD," Sam said.

There are so many of us who do have it. It wasn't until then that I realized Sam had PTSD. I was dismayed because he seemed so happy and balanced. But his wife, Kathy, confirmed that he did, indeed, have problems. They had suffered tough times during their marriage since his return home from Vietnam. I couldn't believe that Sam had PTSD. I had always refused to believe there was such a thing, and I didn't have it either! That is why I titled this book *Invisible*, because PTSD is not a visible injury and is not recognizable to most of us from the outside.

Sam encouraged me to contact the local Vet Center in Sacramento. It was frustrating getting started, but worth the trouble. Once in their system, I was able to start talking, one on one, to a trained counselor. In the beginning, I didn't know what I wanted or needed. I did know that I was not going to start telling this stranger— certified counselor or not—about the thoughts in my head.

I wasn't yet ready to tell some stranger, someone who didn't see combat and was not a part of my brotherhood, about my guilt for the guys who died in Vietnam. I would not reveal thoughts of my own suicide. It would be more than a year of meetings with counselors and psychiatrists— and Sam's encouragement— before I would be ready to talk and to begin to heal.

Unfortunately, my friend Sam, my confidant, died due to prostate and pancreatic cancers. Both cancers are presumptive conditions of Agent Orange poisoning that he got while serving in Vietnam.

Sam Topps died March 3, 2009, and I often think, "I miss you, Sam."

Sergeant Major Sam L. Topps was given a military funeral, which included a twenty-one-gun salute. There were so many people; I felt compelled to go outside the church for a while, even there at my friend's funeral.

Later that day while alone and reflecting, I started to cry, but I found that I was not crying for Sam alone, but also for myself. I cried for all my guilt and anxiety. I even cried out of pride that seemed to wash uncontrollably over me, pride for the honor of knowing Sam and the honor of my country. But it was pride laced with guilt, anxiety, and regret for leaving my fellow combat brothers.

22

And Then!

lthough difficult to watch, *Platoon* is my favorite movie.
It speaks to me. The characters, their fears, and their
actions—I recognize them. Although I had different
experiences in Vietnam, I felt and thought much like the men of
Charlie Company. Sometimes when my wife goes out of town for
an overnight trip to visit her sisters, (which I believe is as much of
an excuse for her to get away from me for a while as it is actually
to visit her sisters), I put my copy in the DVD player and watch
it. On these solitary occasions, I allow myself to give in to my
emotion. Only after watching *Platoon* multiple times did I make
the connection between the characters in that story, their PTSD,
and mine. I wondered how those soldiers had dealt with their
trauma—or if they even had. It was then that I decided to write
my story. The slow healing of my trauma gave me the desire and
ability to convey my experience. I wanted to write my memoir to
bring a better understanding among all who care about PTSD, the
victims, their families, their friends, and those merely interested
in new knowledge.

Others have had it worse. My actions may not have been
all that bad. However, I am a different person than I was before
being sent to war in Vietnam, growing up in Southern California,

innocently chasing girls, and going to the beach. I didn't contest going to war, but it wasn't my choice.

From the time I discharged from the army in September 1969 through August 2010, I worked at thirty-six jobs, an astonishing number over an employment career of forty-one years. The number looms even larger, considering that my employment with the El Dorado County Sheriff's Department as a correctional officer lasted almost ten years. I worked at law enforcement, truck driving, car sales, solar water heater sales, security, and others. Leaving most jobs, I never thought that my exit was for anything more than an unappreciative boss. Looking back and understanding what I now know, I truly believe I was reacting to the stresses and pressures of PTSD. It was my own depression and illogical thought pattern that pushed me beyond the tipping point. I am amazed that my family—or anyone who knows me—has stayed supportive over all these years. My wife Betty is an amazing woman. She has been, not only supportive, but also understanding in everything I have ventured.

Through my many rants, mood swings, and plain-stupid actions, Betty stayed with me. She is my one true love. She and our faith in God the Father, Son, and Holy Spirit have brought me this far. Betty has been my divine gift from God because she has had the tolerance and patience to give me encouragement when I was down and the strength to pull me back up. After each employment fiasco, Betty was there to provide understanding without judgment.

Faith in God is a powerful force. I can't say that I have been given divine guidance every time I have faltered because I didn't always turn to my faith when I was in need. However, when I do pray and put faith in God, circumstances seem tolerable. My son, John; daughter, Tiffany; and granddaughter, Dahlia, all make me a better man. It is because of them that I want to live and to be a person that they enjoy and want to be around.

AFTER ALMOST FORTY YEARS, I was a non-believer in the elusive and invisible PTSD. I went through life, I thought then, without much problem. Sure, I had been through more than thirty different jobs and was in my second marriage, but there was nothing wrong with me. I had a son and daughter who were doing well on their own, plus a beautiful granddaughter. I owned two decent cars and a nice home.

I had heard of PTSD and even come across some guys who said they had it, but I thought they were just a bunch of sniveling, candy asses looking for sympathy and a handout. Eventually, my blinders came off. PSTD was no longer invisible. I finally recognized the many symptoms that plagued me.

Attending the VA's PTSD group sessions helped me to talk about my flashbacks, nightmares, fears, and numbing to personal relationships. I still suffer, of course, but not as often. Now, at least, I can talk to other vets who know and understand what I think and feel. My survivor guilt weighs heavy, and thoughts of suicide plague my mind. So many good young men died, and I did not. Why? I should be there with them. Of course, my daily dose of 200 milligrams Wellbutrin SR helps keep me stable and on track. A low dose of Prazosin keeps away the reoccurring nightmares. I fully understand that I have PTSD, yet I am still uncomfortable telling anyone.

There are many levels of PTSD. For some, the effect is small. Others completely lose the ability to function in daily life. I consider myself reasonably successful in coping and functioning in life, but am clinically categorized with other survivors of PTSD in the fifty-percent category. The Department of Veterans Affairs rates veteran-related PTSD on a scale called the Global Assessment Factor, from zero percent to 100 percent and all ranges in between. A rating of 100 percent on the scale typifies a person who is completely functional, having no symptoms of PTSD. A rating of zero-percent describes a victim totally and utterly unable to care for themselves and unable to function in society.

With the help of doctors and counselors at the Veterans Administration Hospitals and Vet Center counseling, I understand I am not alone in what I think, what I feel, how I act toward others, and how I feel about myself. I now have a better understanding of where I'm at and what I can expect to accomplish. My VA counselors have taught me that, although the scars and traumas of *my* war still exist, I can accept that they are real and allow myself to move on with my life.

POST-TRAUMATIC STRESS IS NOT just an injury of modern wars. It has affected warriors of every war. In an interview between actor Tom Hanks and news anchor Tom Brokaw (both of whom I greatly respect for their talented work, reputation, moral ethics, and philanthropic goals) the pair commented on the opening of a museum dedicated to WWII. They discussed how valiant and courageous the WWII veterans were, and they were correct. They talked about how those veterans came home after the war and went to work, started families, and did what they needed to do, which is mostly correct.

When I heard their statements in this interview, I became enraged. I was pissed off. It is typical of people to ignore the failures of the veterans of World War II and then specifically point to Vietnam vets and accuse them of being deviant, law- breaking, troubled individuals who are putting a dredge on American society. Yes, Vietnam vets have problems, but so did and do everyone else from all other wars. If they want to point a finger, point it at everyone, or not point at all.

A documentary about Vietnam on the History Channel, said WWII infantrymen averaged ten days combat per year, while Vietnam infantrymen endured two-hundred-forty days combat in a year! What an astounding level of violence and trauma for anyone to experience in one year.

What these good-hearted and well-intentioned gentlemen

either did not know, forgot, or perhaps deliberately did not mention, was the high rate of returning veterans from World War II, who came home to become alcoholics, wife batterers, homeless transients, and suicidal. Their statements, rather their omission of statements, rang clear to me that society does not want to disparage the WWII veterans, but are quick to blame and judge how messed up Vietnam veterans are. That may be true, but it is not just the Vietnam veteran. At least we are now getting help!

I WAS HAUNTED FOR MANY YEARS BY TWO particular recurring nightmares. They repeated nearly twice per week. After unsuccessfully trying to explain my dreams to my psychiatrist, I thought that I would try to draw pictures of my dreams. I drew a single picture for each dream to help me identify and explain the basic layout of them to my psychiatrist.

As it turned out, drawing the two pictures helped me to cope with regular daily life. I later found out that it is a therapeutic assignment to have patients draw out their dreams, fears, or emotions, or whatever is bothering them. I think that because I was concentrating on the dreams during the daytime, it was allowing my brain to rest at night. I started sleeping a little better. I did not wake up as often. When I did wake up, it wasn't in a panic anymore. I still have dreams, but thanks to medication, not my reoccurring nightmares, at least not as frequently or as intense.

In the first dream, I find myself walking in a wooded area. I see lots of undergrowth with dried leaves and broken twigs and branches on the ground. A stream runs through the middle. Sometimes it has water flowing, but most of the time, it is dry or just slightly muddy. The trees are deep dark-green to a light yellow-green, reminiscent of turning fall leaves. Often I can hear the dry leaves crushing under my feet. Other times it is quiet. In some episodes, I walk in both directions, but more often I walk just in one direction.

I never cross over to the other side of the stream. Getting to the other side appears difficult, but possible by climbing up the bank and onto an old tree log lying at an angle from the top of the bank and down to the edge of the stream. The other side is a dark, thick, tall forest. It is so thickly forested that I can only see into it a couple of trees deep. Much like the darkness of a canopied jungle, it is so thick that the earth below is virgin to the sun's light.

I don't know if I am afraid to cross over or if it is just too heavily wooded to walk there. Sometimes this dream is calm, and I am just walking. Sometimes I am trying to get away or sense that I am being stalked. Sometimes I feel that I am the hunter or that I am stalking something. A few times, I have been carrying an M16. One time when walking in the less-traveled direction, I came into a clearing of the woods and into my other recurring dream, connecting the two dreams together.

My second dream finds me returning to Vietnam for a second tour of duty. I arrive at a location with new and improved Dusters. I am in a small apartment kitchen, talking to a couple of my new crew members.

One of them says, "Come on. I'll show you the guns."

I get up and see a ladder on the wall. It is vertical, like one that might be on a submarine or ship. Climbing the ladder, we come into the turret of the same old Dusters I was on before. I look around and see a large graded-off hill. It is that same old stinking red dirt. As I look around, six Dusters are spaced in various locations on the hill. Sometimes this dream starts in a kitchen, sometimes in the turret, and other times I am standing back, looking at the whole area like a spectator.

From the turret of the guns, I look out over a field of tall elephant grass, sprinkled with a few trees that have dry or broken branches burned or scarred from battle. Some are fully foliated, but most are dead and have been destroyed by the destruction of our guns' exploding ammunition. It is at the far end of this field and on the left side where I entered into this area and look up toward the Dusters on the graded hill just as I had seen in my first recurring dream.

No matter how this dream starts, it always ends the same. At some point in the dream, I see movement in the tall grass, far off in the field and to the left. As I watch, I can tell that the movement comes by way of villagers dressed in black pajamas. They wear large cone-shaped, basket-woven hats. When they get closer, I see that they are carrying rifles and starting to crouch down and take cover as if to make themselves a smaller target. I start repeatedly yelling, "Fire." No one is there or doing anything. I am alone. As I start to be overrun, (a term used to define when the enemy has infiltrated or broken through the perimeter) I wake up, in panic mode.

IT IS 0313. I CAREFULLY PUSH DOWN THE COVERS and roll out of bed in one smooth motion without disturbing Betty. In the darkness, my eyes are at full night vision and able to detect the slightest bit of light coming through the bedroom window or from the digital clock on the kitchen stove reflecting through the open bedroom door. In my effort to maintain silence and stealth, I remain barefoot. I consciously avoid the small piece of plastic runner Betty had put on the floor near the bedroom entry and step onto the tile that runs through the kitchen, dining area, and front entry. I am up for my regular perimeter check, walking through the house in the dark, on guard duty, checking doors and windows. It is May; the early morning temperature is cool.

I look through the small beveled, leaded glass window in the front door through a spot that allows me an undistorted view of the yard and street. I see the small branches of nearby trees slightly moving in a gentle breeze. I feel the coolness of the glass against my face. The neighbor two doors down and across the street has left his porch light on again three nights in a row. Next, I move to a dining room window, pulling back the shade just enough to allow me to see if anything is up close. Satisfied that it is clear, I open the shade enough to expose a clear view.

A black and white cat belonging to another neighbor is stalking something in the honeysuckle near the front porch. Briefly, the street is lit up from headlights; the car turns at the corner and does not pass by. The cat gives up its hunt and trots back across the street.

I think about three of my fellow PTSD group brothers and feel a need to call and check on one of them, the marine. I resist the urge, telling myself that even though he is most likely also up pacing through his home, checking his own perimeter, I should wait until a more normal hour to phone. I fight back the thought that he might be in need, that something may have happened. I note the time, 0401.

I hear water flowing in the pipes; the sprinkler has started to water the front yard. I look out the front window to confirm the sprinkler is, indeed, on. The time is 0403, which means the timer is three minutes slow because it was set to come on at 0400. I went to bed last night at 2315, probably got to sleep about 2335, slept until 0310. That is three hours, thirty-five minutes sleep before I woke for guard duty. I decide to go back to bed and sleep until about 0745. It is Sunday, and I can sleep in. We won't leave for church until 10:30: I'll call Bart in the morning.

"Dear Lord, please protect him, and give him your peace," I pray.

I HOPE CUBA, LEONARD, AND DENNIS ARE OK.

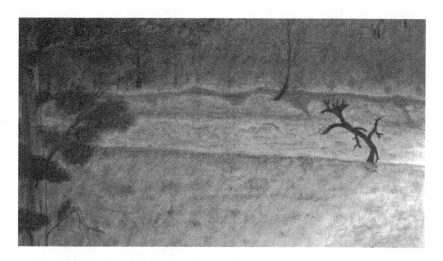

Dream number one: In the forest with creek bed

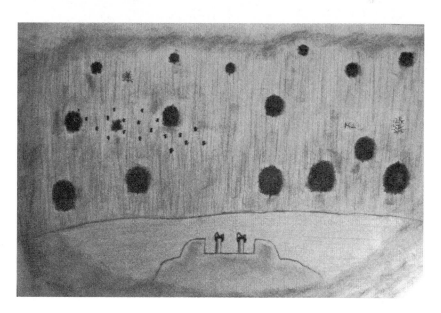

Dream number two: VC advancing on Blaylock's position

23

Is This a Dream or Reality?

An image of the globe appears. The United States of America as seen from space fills my computer screen because I had typed "Google Earth" in the search window of my web browser. I found the program, agreed without reading the terms and conditions of use, and waited for it to install.

At the "Google Earth" home page, there is a fly-to box. I type in the name of my hometown, Covina, California. The globe comes forward and turns. Rotating toward the West Coast of the United States it zooms in on the town of Covina.

"Wow, this is cool!" I think.

I am looking at the rooftops of the town where I grew up. I figure out how to zoom down to street level and move the cursor to view the street from different angles. I recognize other streets and buildings.

Covina has changed in the forty-three years since I left, but not so much that I cannot recognize the streets where I rode my bike and the house where I grew up. A tall tree grows in the front yard now. It wasn't there when I was growing up, and the current resident has a motor home parked in the driveway. There are swimming pools in the backyards of a lot more homes that most people could not afford back then. The trees are full-grown and now mature. It looks like some new buildings have replaced old ones, but for the most part, Covina hasn't changed much.

The elementary school is still right across the street. I look down at its classroom buildings and remember Peggy, my second-grade girlfriend. She pestered me, always wanting to play marriage or wedding. It seemed to me we were always walking-down-the-aisle. When we stopped at the end of a short arm-in-arm stroll, she would say some words, pull me toward her for a kiss, and then announce, "OK, we're married!" Then, we would run off to play hide-n-seek.

One year Peggy had a birthday party at the municipal pool, the Covina City Plunge. She pulled me under the water, and we kissed. I laugh to myself remembering the look on her father's face when we rose to the surface, and he stood at the edge of the pool looking down at me.

I return to the screen, scrolling left. I find Covina High School.

"This is really cool," I repeat to myself. I feel excitement at what I am seeing.

"What should I search next?"

I type my current address, and the globe blurs, rotates, and comes into position directly over my home. An X marks the spot. I zoom in. Our house is clearly displayed in detail. I see our corner lot, the crosswalk for children walking to and from school. The trees are in full foliage, and it looks as if I might have recently mowed the lawn.

THE HOUSE IS QUIET. MY WIFE BETTY is watching television in the next room; I am alone in the office.

Amazed at what Google Earth can do, I type in Fort Lewis,

Washington. I feel my body tense a bit. I shipped out from Fort Lewis in 1968 to go to Vietnam. The globe rotates to the north and zooms in on Fort Lewis. I type in Seattle Tacoma Airport, and the globe rotates a short distance north.

"I can chart my military journey!"

My flight to Vietnam stopped in Japan to refuel, so I typed in Osaka, Japan. The globe rotates again over the Pacific Ocean and comes to rest on the island nation of Japan. Fully engrossed in this new tool, I type in a new location, Cam Ranh Bay, Vietnam. This time, as the globe on the screen begins to turn and zoom in on the location, I feel an increasing apprehension that quickens my pulse. I take deep, heavy breaths, but I want to go on. The globe zooms in close enough to the earth that it has become a map rather than the globe. Hesitating slightly at each keystroke, I type in Da Nang, Vietnam, and the map moves again to the north, up the coast of Vietnam to the coastal town of Da Nang.

The anxiety is real now. My pulse races faster still. My heart is pounding hard inside my chest; my gut is tight; my throat is dry. I have a feeling like something might jump out at me from around a blind corner, yet I felt compelled to continue. This time I type in the location Dong Ha, Vietnam. The map moves a bit to the north and identifies an area about eight miles west from the coast as being Dong Ha, Vietnam. My palms are sweaty now as I look at the screen, and then type Rockpile, Vietnam.

The map moves to the left, following a yellow line on the surface labeled "9." I can tell that it is identifying what was Highway 9. I feel goose bumps on my neck, and my whole body begins to shake as if gripped by a frigid Arctic wind. I read the words on the pointer: "Rockpile, 1967/68."

I continue to stare at the monitor, but I am no longer staring at an image on the computer screen. I am there.

I AM STANDING OUTSIDE THE BUNKER on OP Ben, the Duster parked behind me, and I am looking out at the forested hills of the Central Highlands. I see Camp Rockpile below and to the left the Rockpile, a single mountain of almost solid stone, rising up out of the earth and standing alone as if it were a monument to the land. There is the cave I use for target practice. The red dirt road snakes its way through the valley below, moving from Da Nang on the eastern coast, across this narrowest part of the entire country, past Khe Sanh, all the way to the western border and on into Laos.

I am taken back forty-two years. I see Leonard, Dennis, and Cuba, and my heart pulls toward them. I see the marine in the poncho raise his right arm to show me that his hand is barely attached. I see Lan, the Vietnamese boy. Tears swell in my eyes, the muscles in my jaw tighten, and my teeth dig into my lower lip. My breath is labored, deep, and slow. I stare at the monitor, shaking quietly as tears fill my eyes.

Other than the markings on the map, the image reveals no evidence that a war was ever fought there. Areas along the river are marked as fishing villages. Using the zoom, I can see buildings. Roads that were just dirt and gravel when I was there are now paved.

After a time, I think I have composed myself, and I call to my wife, "Betty, come look at this."

She walks into the room. Looking not at the computer, but at me, she asks, "Are you OK?"

"Look at this," I say, nodding my head toward the computer monitor. She does not understand what she is seeing, so, with tears again and a quiver in my voice, I tell her, "That's where I was for a year in Vietnam."

She puts her arms around me and stands beside me as I stare at the screen in mournful silence.

I think, "I am getting better, but unlike me, the jungle is completely healed."

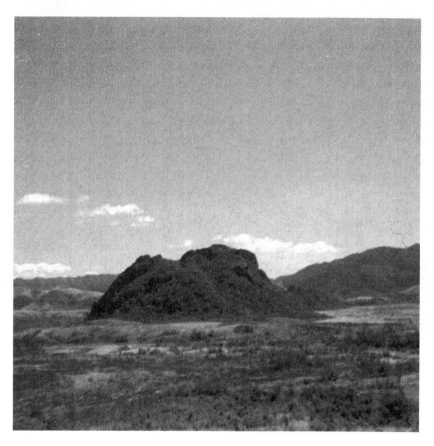

The Rockpile

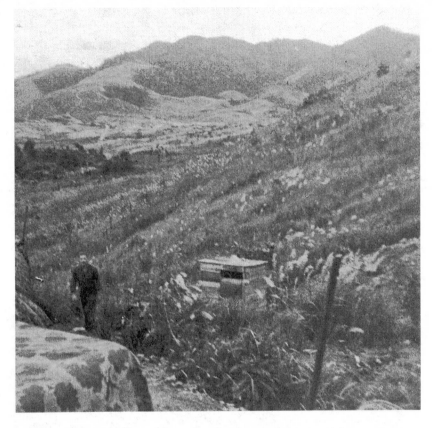

Leonard with Camp Rockpile in the background

24

Getting Better

L etting go! That's easier said than done and not just a cliché. Quite possibly, healing from PTSD is much like quitting smoking or drinking. First, a person has to want to get better. A victim can either accept or reject the help given by family, friends, the Vet Center and VA Counselors, but those who suffer must be ready and desire to say good-bye to their demons and fears.

I have good days and bad. I can see that, as with all things in life, the more I practice something, the better I get at it. Now I must continue to practice what I have learned at the VA. I must let go and realize that my success is being shown in the span of time between lapses. Perhaps the word *practice* is not the best word to use, but for me, practice is in the attempt to smile when I don't actually feel like it. Practice may be telling a war story to someone who is not a psych counselor, but a curious person who simply wants to know. Practice, for me, is going places where there are a lot of people or strangers. Practice is not standing with my back to the wall, but actually mingling with the group. In the beginning, I may have gone only one day when I did not think about my experiences and go into a depression. Now I go days and sometimes a week or more without relapsing into depression and having thoughts of the war.

I reflect on Vietnam when I meet with my fellow veterans at scheduled VA meetings, but with each incremental meeting, the exhaustion is not as severe. It is not as upsetting as it was in the beginning. I am learning how to allow myself the opportunity to explore beyond my comfort zone. Before I started counseling, I was not willing to talk to anyone about Vietnam or what I did and saw there. Even among fellow veterans, we would usually just make general statements and affirm each other. That did not require us to confess or divulge anything that we weren't willing to tell. On a personal level, I now enjoy people whom I would not have spent time with just a couple of years ago.

Just two years ago, I would not have been able to talk to the people I care about, let alone write about my experience or feelings. I have gotten better, not just in being able to write my story, but in my ability to go out with my wife and enjoy people. I still have times when I don't want to hang around long, so I just start telling people goodnight and make my way to the door. However, the whole purpose is that I am becoming increasingly tolerant of the things that for a very, very long time were my shortcomings. I am getting my life back.

Dr. Melinda Keenan explained PTSD to me. Drawing a heart on the display board, she said, "This is what our heart looked like before going to Vietnam."

Then she draws a squiggly line across one edge of the heart. "After seeing your first dead body, you get a little tear." She draws another squiggly line. "After that, the first time you were shot at."

She draws another crooked line on the heart and says, "You see one of your squad members get his legs blown off from a mine or booby trap."

She draws yet another line on the heart.

"Then, during a firefight, your buddy gets hit and dies right there next to you, or maybe even in your arms."

Another long squiggly line goes across the heart. Now the heart is full of lines indicating tears, each one representing a trauma.

"Now," she says, "you came back home and managed to keep the heart beating even though there was blood loss. What we here at the VA are trying to do is to stitch up all those tears on your heart."

She draws little stitch marks across all the squiggly lines that she had drawn on the heart. "Your heart," she says, "will never be new again. The scars will always be there just like any external wound in life, but now you can start to heal. When the wounds are stitched, the healing can begin! Now, when we look at the heart, we see it with stitches where the tears were. We can't make the heart new again, but we can stitch it back together so that it can heal. The scars are still there, but it is whole and in one piece so that it can more properly function."

I WILL ADD TO HER STORY SAYING, even though the heart is sutured and healing, that does not mean there will not be an occasional skipped beat or an arrhythmia, but the best part is that it is still working. I relate my healing of PTSD to that of alcoholism. Once you have been an alcoholic, you are always an alcoholic even though you do not drink any more. For PTSD, it is much the same. Once you have PTSD, you will always have it. The healing and therapy allow a victim to understand and cope with the symptoms in a positive way, but the disease is still there.

My tears, rips, and scars are for the wounded marine we took to an LZ for medevac; for the other marines we weren't able to save or get to in time; for the marine I abandoned by not answering his letter; for Lan, the young Vietnamese boy; for every thought I had that I would die in that forsaken place; and for all my fellow brothers I left there. Of course, I remember the first time I knew that I had been shot at, seeing dead bodies, both the enemy and ours, but without a doubt, my greatest trauma is survivors' guilt. Why did I come home when so many good and deserving young men died instead of me? I often wish that I had died there too! It would have all been so much easier.

My VA counseling group for PTSD culminated with the writing of a letter. It can address a specific person, named or unnamed, or to no particular individual at all. The letters are written with the intent of expressing sorrow, remorse, guilt, anger, or, for any reason that gets to the core of the writer's trauma. While participating in this group, I wrote three letters. The last one generated the most discussion in the group and during discussion turned to what I thought a profound understanding of my reason for the letter. My three letters are included here; the last one follows with the groups' response.

PTSD Letter to Lan

Monday, September 14, 2009

Dear Lan,

  I sincerely hope you are doing well.

  You may not remember me, but I certainly remember you. You made quite an impression on me. I was on a tank crew; there were five of us, and we all thought you were quite special. We met you some time in 1968; you were only eight years old. You smoked as many cigarettes a day as any of us did; back then no one thought about it being bad for our health—we just thought it was funny to see such a young kid smoking. But what the hell, you had been through so much already that smoking was the least of your problems.

  To refresh your memory, when I met you, I was with my fellow crew members and Duster, parked on a ridge overlooking the Song Cam Lo River. We were there to provide security for a Seabee's unit that was getting rock to help make better roads in the area. Since the Seabees were working at the water's edge, this location gave us a good firing capability to both sides and up and down the river. No one ever crossed to the north side of the river because that was Charlie's!

We had been at this location for about a week when one day you just walked up the path toward us. While still a little way out, you said, "Hey GI, you number one." We were pretty sure you weren't concealing any weapons because the only thing you were wearing was a torn pair of pants.

It wasn't long before we all trusted each other. We made sure that you had food each day and a few extra smokes to get you through the night. You said that your village was about a mile west of our location, wherever that was!

After a short time of getting to know you, you told us what had happened to you and your family. I do not know how long it had been from when it happened to when we met, but I believe that it had been about a year.

You told us that VC had come to your village trying to get the villagers to join and aid their cause. Your parents did not cooperate. In retaliation, they then raped and killed your older sister while forcing you all to watch. Still resisting, you were also beaten and forced to watch while they murdered your parents by decapitation. They then left you there to die. Fortunately, you were saved, thanks to other villagers.

Now, we never tried to confirm your story, but true or false, either way, I guess that deep inside it gave us hope that we were doing something good there.

I didn't think about it then, but given that we were in

the mountains, I guess that you are Hmong, or what we called Montagnard.

For such a young kid, you seemed to know a lot, about what was going on. It wasn't long into our relationship that you began telling us when you had seen more activity in your area. I'm not positive about this, but I think I remember you telling us that if there ever was a day that you did not come see us, we should be extra careful. There wasn't a day when you did not show up, but when you were there, we never had any problems!

I still think of the way I felt about you and that I thought I could bring you home with me to give you a better life. I told you one time that I wanted to adopt you and take you to America, but you said, "No GI, you go you home, I stay mine."

I look at the pictures of you and me and pray that you survived the war, not only in your home and country, but also in your heart and mind. You understandably had a deep and lasting hatred for your own countrymen who did such terrible things to their own people.

It is terribly unfortunate how humans can be so vile and corrupt toward their own mankind. To try to pass it off as "human nature" seems so obscene and trivial.

There is just not a worthy explanation for actions taken by any person in a time of war, a time when hatred becomes the norm and morality is replaced by cunning deceit: when the mantra becomes, "how much can I hurt them." What a waste it becomes; hatred between people, instead of compassion.

Lan, I am writing this not because I am asking forgiveness, but because of the loss I still feel for you. You were just a child, and really, so was I. It has been forty-one years since I was in your homeland, and I still live "in" it almost every day.

I pray for your well-being and offer you peace.

Sincerely, GI Bill

Monday, October 26, 2009

Dear Marines,

I am sorry for so many things in my life, but this letter and confronting you have taken me far too long. I don't know your names or faces, but that does not take away the guilt and shame I feel, or the respect I pledge to you.

In June, 1968, you were in an ambush, and were wounded or killed. Two Dusters plus air support were called to help with getting you guys out. I was the gunner on the track in front. I remember seeing your bodies lying in the road ahead of us as we drove in.

We had to drive into position to put out enough fire to allow your fellow marines the opportunity to retrieve other dead, wounded, and surviving marines. Our order was to drive straight in while putting out suppression fire all the way in. To do that meant that we had to drive over your bodies to get into position.

I am so very sorry for having to do what we did to you. I cannot imagine the incredibly intense pain you suffered along with the devastating desecration to your bodies.

In the over forty-one years since then, there have not been many days that go by that you are not remembered and revered. I cry for your loss and hail your dedication to "Duty, Honor, and Country." We were all scared of dying there that day. Many times, I wish that it had been me instead, or that at least we had all died together.

My solace is that you and your fellow marines were not left behind and that God has a better plan. I try to believe that if it were not for you losing your life, there would have been a great many more dead that day, in that place.

I pray for your peace and that we will meet whole someday in Heaven.

Most Sincerely,

Your, Mournful Brother in Arms.

Friday, February 04, 2011

Dear Marine,

I am writing this letter to you today—over forty years late!

I am asking for your forgiveness for two things. First, and most importantly, for not writing back to you after I got your letter from Vietnam. Two; I cannot remember your name or the names of your other squad members. I do not know if it is because of time, or if I buried it away, deep in my mind to avoid the memory.

I believe that I didn't write back to you when I should have because back then I was in denial. That is no excuse, or at least, a lousy one. I think that, at the time, for me the war was over. I did not want to think about it, and I didn't want to return by writing a letter. I couldn't bear going back "there" again! I know that was pretty "chicken shit," but I just couldn't make myself face that again, not even in my mind by writing a letter to you. I am writing you now because of the help I have received from VA counselors and programs.

You certainly needed to hear back from someone you thought "understood," and you definitely needed to have my support, encouragement, and "get well" wishes. I am so ashamed of myself.

When I got your letter, I had been home from "Nam" about a week. My wife and I were visiting my parent's at their home. We had been there just a few minutes when my mom handed me a sealed letter and said it had come for me.

You started your letter by saying that you were writing while lying in a hospital on the coast in Da Nang. You had been wounded with shrapnel in your leg. You said that it wasn't too bad and that you would be returning to your company in a few days.

You told me that your squad had been in the bush on a "seek and destroy" mission. You were about two clicks south of the DMZ and northwest of our old position at "The Rockpile." Your team had been out for three days when NVA hit you in an ambush with grenades, rockets, and AK-47s. You and one other guy were the only survivors from your whole squad.

"They're dead! They're all fucking dead!" I said out loud, dropping my head in my hands as I began to cry.

I remember looking up at Mom, Dad, and my wife. They were just sitting there in silence with a shocked look on their faces. They must have been afraid to say or do anything. I tried to control my sobbing. Wiping my tears, I said something like, "I'm sorry" and got up to go to the kitchen to get a drink of water.

Dad followed me and just stood there next to me with his arm around my shoulders. He didn't say anything; he just stood there with me.

I said, "They're dead; they're all dead," as I started to cry again.

After that, no one ever said anything about it again, and that was the last time I cried for a long, long time.

I am so very sorry,

Bill "Semper Fi, Marine"

AFTER READING THIS LAST letter aloud, I listened to responses from the group. The comments showed sympathy and understanding for my not responding to my friend in Vietnam.

Then Andy, said, "You know, when I got back, it wasn't so good. People didn't like us for being in Vietnam. Nobody even talked about it. If it were me having to write back to a buddy, I don't know that I would have had anything good to say. How could I have written him back and told him that everything had changed. It isn't what I thought it would be when I got home."

There was a sudden realization of truth in the group. Heads bobbed up and down in full agreement as we looked around the room at each other. The feeling that I was not alone and that others felt the same way I did was comforting. It did not mean that I am not troubled, just that I am not the only one. It is a shame that we all felt that way after returning home to the very things that we had longed for the whole time we were gone. Nevertheless, sometimes that's just the way it is!

CONTACTING THE VET Center was the beginning of my journey back to myself.

25

Addendum

I think that I have been reasonably successful in life, in spite of my many job changes. Like everyone, I have had successes and failures. For some of those failures, I've beat myself up; for others, not so much.

I wonder if it is accurate to say that, in the beginning as a youth, I was given an attitude of presumptive expectation of a good life merely by growing up in sunny Southern California. After all, when my father moved us to California from Mississippi, it was with the intention of having a better life. The saying was, "Go West, Young Man," and a lot of the nation did just that in the next few years following the Second World War. People left cold, wet climates and hot, dry lands to go to California where there were orange groves, prosperity, and belief in a better tomorrow. I believe that each of us is a product of our environment, not just the households where we are raised. Each of us is also influenced by the location and attitude of our entire zone of existence and nurturing.

There are Vietnam veterans who had different experiences and would, therefore, give a different account of what they saw and felt, but the trauma that causes their PTSD is their own and is deep within. You may ask why are some affected by PTSD, and not others. Why doesn't everyone have PTSD? Some may say that it is because those inflicted had a more caring heart or maybe they were mentally weaker. I do not know the answer, but I surmise that it has nothing to do with either of those opinions. Rather I believe it is simply that we are all individuals. Just as we all have different fingerprints, eye retina, and DNA, we are all susceptible to effects of traumatic events that occur in our lives.

Some were OK for a while. Some were OK for a long time. Some felt it right away, but most feel it at some time or another. Some were weak; some were strong. Some were brave; most were scared. All were represented there.

Some found solace in alcohol, some with drugs, and some with both. Some found it in a career, abandoning everything and everyone to be a workaholic. Some of us just dropped out. Some dropped out just for a while and others permanently. Some of us learned to suppress it, pushing it down into a deep, dark place to allow cobwebs to grow over it. Some found that the only way to kill the enemy within was to kill the one that carried the enemy—themselves. In fact, suicide is high among Vietnam vets. I know I have thought about it. After all, what is the use of dealing with all the "BS"? Nothing's going to change anyway. Just let the world go on without me.

Some were industrious and made a name for themselves. Some became public servants, and some wasted away into anonymity. Some became wealthy, and some were destitute. All just did what they could to survive. In the end, it was just about survival, never knowing that we were holding or harboring compressed thoughts and feelings and the trouble it would bring.

I think that most of us who felt it right away tended to choose alcohol or drugs. A lot of us found other ways to cope. Some even found the ability to hate with such intensity that they stayed to fight and kill for as long as they could by returning for multiple tours. That way, they could deny having feelings or problems until forced to face them when returning to civilization. Not that everyone who stayed for multiple tours had that intensity of hate, but it was an excellent "out" for those who did. These problems are the result of the emotions of fear, betrayal, loss, guilt, and rejection from our families, friends, and country.

I HAVE BEEN BACK TO GOOGLE EARTH many times since that first experience, and each time I return to that location it is difficult, but not like the first time. It is still painful, but it lessens each time, and I don't get the same intense emotions.

The memories told here are mine, and mine alone. There are many other memories and traumas still waiting to be told.

No matter how varied or complex the trauma, the effect and aftermath for the veteran are the same. We all suffer from trauma and terrible events in life, but if it were not for the United States military veteran, standing at the wall, defending our country's freedoms, this and many other stories could not have been told.

Thank you to our current veterans. You have the torch. Carry it the best you can, with honor and pride.

God be with you and grant you peace.

LYING IN BED ONE NIGHT while particularly restless, and unable to sleep, I started to pray. I was praying silently with my thoughts to God. I prayed, "I am thankful for our country and military, and I'm asking God's Holy Spirit to protect our troops and return them home safely to their families and loved ones, and the things that are important to them. I pray for God's guidance and blessing on my writing."

During my prayer, I believe that I received an answer, or message from God. There was no loud thunderous voice from above; it was more like a thought. But rather than coming from within my mind, it seemed to come to me from outside my mind. The message told me, "This work is my purpose, God's plan for me: that I may help others in their search for peace and understanding in their life."

I now pray that after reading *Invisible* you have received the understanding and knowledge that will guide you to find the peace you deserve.

Invisible

Sources for Help

V et Centers offer a wealth of help for veterans suffering with PTSD, as well as other veterans, who have returned from armed hostility and can benefit from counseling, outreach, and referrals to help them with the readjustment to civilian life.

The program was born in 1979 when Congress realized that a significant number of Vietnam-era vets were experiencing readjustment problems, including PTSD. Today more than 300 Vet Centers operate under the jurisdiction of the U.S. Department of Veterans Affairs. In many cases, families of returning veterans are also eligible for services from local Vet Centers.

To find a location near you, look in your local phone book under the United States government pages or access the Internet and visit www.va.gov/directory/guide to search for a location in your area.

The Vet Center has a great slogan: "It takes the courage and strength of a warrior to ask for help."

The U.S. Department of Veterans Affairs also operates a network of hospitals and medical care facilities organized in twenty-three geographic areas across the United States. If you served in the active military service and were separated under any condition other than "dishonorable," you may qualify for VA health care benefits. Vets who meet minimum service requirements or who fall under a category of enhanced eligibility can receive medical services. The first step is to apply. Use the Internet to access www.va.gov/healthbenefits/apply. Be prepared to show proof of service (DD214) at these facilities when checking in your first time.

If you have an immediate need for help, feel helpless and suffer from thoughts of suicide, immediately seek assistance and care. Don't wait. One of the first places you can call now is the National Suicide Prevention Lifeline. It is available nationwide, twenty-four hours a day. Call 1-800-273-8255 and press "1" for veterans.